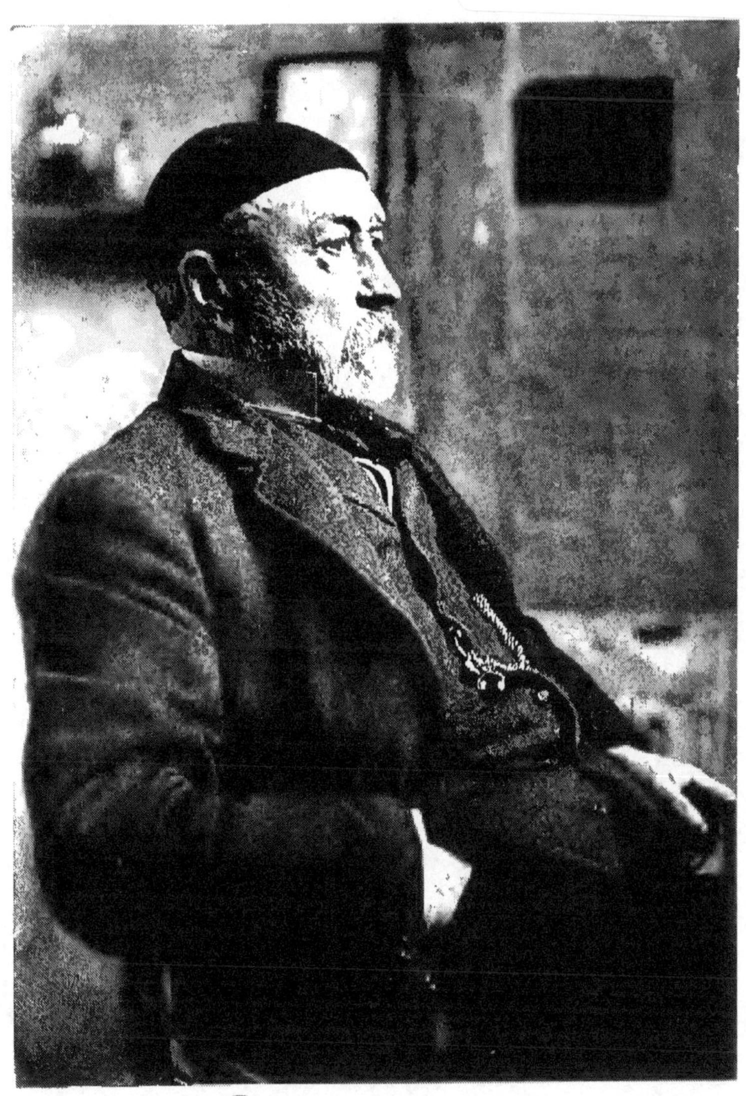

T. Armstrong

THOMAS ARMSTRONG, C.B.

A MEMOIR

1832–1911

LONDON
MARTIN SECKER
NUMBER FIVE JOHN STREET
ADELPHI
MCMXII

PREFATORY NOTE

The friends of Thomas Armstrong were anxious to mark their appreciation of the place he held in their estimations, and a privately circulated memoir was one of the means proposed as a tribute to his memory. The nucleus was to consist of the reminiscences written during his later years, in which are set forth his early Paris experiences and the growth of his friendships there. With consideration the idea grew, and it was decided to publish a short biography and to reproduce some of his work. It was hoped that Mr. William De Morgan might be induced to write the book, but his own literary engagements prevented his undertaking any fresh work, though the following letter, written to Mrs. Armstrong, shows his sympathy with the venture. The task therefore fell into the hands of several friends to whom Mrs. Armstrong has rendered signal service, by her advice, information, and revision. Miss Eleanor Rowe collected, with great care and a labour most willingly given, the official record, from which the notes after 1881 have been mostly drawn, and into my all too inexperienced hands fell the editing of the whole material. As regards the illustrations, to the reader unfamiliar with Armstrong's original work it should be stated that it is almost impossible to render its charm in reproduction. The beauty and harmony of his compositions, together with his delicate sense of colour, prove elusive when mechanically expressed.

L. M. LAMONT.

LETTER FROM
MR. WILLIAM DE MORGAN

127, Church Street,
Chelsea, S.W.

24th August, 1912

DEAR MRS. ARMSTRONG,

I am afraid any "reminiscences" of your husband from my pen will make but a poor show. For the truth is that though I have a long and affectionate recollection of him, it does not afford any such detailed memories as resolve themselves into narratives. When we met, our conversation turned on the applied arts—on Persian tiles and Gubbio dishes—much too technical to be remembered or chronicled.

Nevertheless I actually knew him before '72, forty years ago! Because I burned the roof off number 40 Fitzroy Square in that year, and it was from that house I went (with I forget whom) to pay a visit to "Tom Armstrong" in Charlotte Street. All I remember of this incident of a remote past is that he had painted a girl in a tree, and did not like her place in the picture, so thought of repainting her on the other side of the tree —and I believe did so, later. My introducer (whose name and identity have taken flight from my mind) said that this was "Armstrong's method." I thought it a bad method, as it involved the sacrifice of the first figure; and that in this case was very regrettable.

I remember further that we went round—all we, like sheep—to Albert Moore's studio, somewhere between the two houses, and found him painting young ladies dressed in white and lilac *nocturnes*, and I think playing battledore and shuttlecock. I can verify nothing.

Not long after this followed my conflagration in Fitzroy Square. I fled to Chelsea and incubated tiles and pots in a back garden with a mulberry tree in it. This went on for a while—Time existed then, I know; but, as for its length, "Good faith, I am no wiser than a daw!" Another epoch followed, attended by more pots, at another house a few doors off—now replaced by a Roman church—and in this house I recall the fact of many visits from your husband, but cannot particularise them. I can recollect his coming to my crockery shop with Mr. and Mrs. George Howard, and I am able to fix the date of this as just before the dinner-party at their house, mentioned at p. 41 of the Memoir.

I *think* that I owed him some of my introduction to Leighton, though I don't exactly know how much. I however gratefully ascribe to him an exercise of good-will towards my imperfect ceramics resulting in other opportunities than that supplied by the *hiatus valde deflendi* (I hope that's right) on the walls of the Arab Hall. Needless to say, no such advancement of the pottery business could command the gratitude due for a small share of Leighton—small, though above my deserts. For the slightest acquaintance with the President was a revelation of one of the most brilliant personalities of his time, and one which no acquaintance with his pictures can possibly supply.

It is much to be rejoiced at that your husband wrote his recollections of the *Trilby* period in Paris. Every scrap of a memory of the author of *Peter Ibbetson* is a thing to be preserved—indeed, a thing whose loss would be lamentable. For that novel is certainly the greatest achievement of romantic pathos—or should we say pathetic romance—that our time has seen. Its individuality intersects with that of nothing I know in fiction. It turns up ground untouched by the ploughshares of even Dickens and Thackeray. After reading it, years after, the mere names he chose for his characters ring into one's heart like phrases of music.

I knew him very little, and would it had been otherwise! As far as the chances of time and place go it might have been, for in 1860 or '61 I occupied a first-floor front studio in Newman Street. There I pretended to be a Painter. The back room was the den of a young artist who sang French songs all day. It was not, I believe, his own studio, but a friend's. When this friend turned up, which he generally did, the noise and laughter, the lulls for comic anecdotes and the outbursts that followed, the suggestions of capsized furniture and chases round the room—well! they were what I have heard described as a *caution!* When the actual occupant was alone, he made no more noise than went with the singing of an enjoyable selection of French songs; I think the *Sieur de Framboisy* was a favourite.

The young man in possession was du Maurier, and the visiting landlord was Whistler. But never a word did I interchange with either, and though I met du Maurier later, it was not above half-a-dozen times all told. My only very vivid recollection of him shows me the inside of a railway carriage, and himself and a friend (probably Harold Power) singing duets from *Cox and Box* into the ears of *my*self and a friend, and the rattle of the train making hay of the music. I was coming back from a visit to Stoke-on-Trent with Horatio Lucas. I never had a merrier or shorter railway journey in my life, and I don't suppose he had. *Cox and Box* had been performed at Manchester, so it was, I think, in 1868.

I cannot add a single Whistler anecdote, unless it be a little characteristic turn of speech about a piece of my crockery. A friend asked his opinion about a dish I had decorated with "ruby lustre." He turned it about—so my friend told me: I was not there—and presently said: "Ought one to forgive a plate because of a peculiar shine?" I could not say at this length of time whether this was a pardonable plate or otherwise. But I feel that a peculiar epigrammatic shine is discernible in the use of the word "forgive," and for its sake am grateful for an adverse criticism, with forgiveness if any is called for.

Which of us will that stern judge, Posterity, forgive. The Author of *Peter Ibbetson* is the horse I put my money on. But each of us will in his degree await judgment at the bar of Posterity. May we all be as fortunate in the witnesses for character as the subject of your memoir

And please do you forgive this rambling letter.

Always yours truly,

WM. DE MORGAN.

CONTENTS

LIST OF ILLUSTRATIONS

MEMOIR

1832 – 1880

THOMAS ARMSTRONG, C.B.

THOMAS ARMSTRONG was born in Manchester, 19 October, 1832. He was the eldest son of Thomas Armstrong, connected with the cotton industry in that city. The family belonged to the Border country, and came to Manchester from Newcastle. His mother was Sarah, youngest daughter of Thomas Evans, of Staleybank, Ashton-under-Lyne, by his marriage with Sarah Savile, of Oldham, by whom he had several children. As the name implies, the family was originally Welsh, and connected some generations back with the Carnarvonshire branch of the Wynnes. The father of Thomas Evans died young, so he and his sister were adopted by his uncle, the Rev. Thomas Evans, D.D., who was subsequently Prebend and Archdeacon of Worcester. Armstrong received his education at a private school at Tarvin in Cheshire, and with a few of his class-mates he kept in touch for many years. He frequently spent his holidays with his mother's sisters, the Misses Evans, who lived at Staleybank, an old-fashioned country house not far from Staleybridge. It is no longer in existence. A man there, known as "owd" Ned Godley, probably a retired keeper, was a source of immense interest to the boy, and he eagerly gleaned knowledge from his stores of information, both of human and natural history, conveyed in the strong Lancashire dialect. Owd Ned would be didactic at times, and say: "I dunnot know much 'bout religion, Tom, but tha' mun ha' *conduct.*"

Staleybank contained many beautiful specimens of china, fine linen, and silver left by Mrs. Armstrong's great-uncle, the archdeacon, who died in 1815. He indubitably possessed excellent taste in such matters as well as a large share of worldly wisdom, and besides the objects themselves he probably bequeathed an appreciation of beauty to his great-great-nephew. Some of the pieces of china were so especially treasured by the aunts that Tom christened them the "sacred vessels of the Temple," and was probably scolded for want of respect towards these household gods. He was full of pranks, and in a diary kept by one of the aunts is the sentence: "Tom is a clever boy, but is a very naughty one."

In the attics of Staleybank were hair-trunks and boxes full of costumes of the end of the eighteenth and beginning of the nineteenth centuries, which in later years were much used by Armstrong in his pictures. They most probably influenced his choice, as he seemed to turn naturally to that period.

School ended early in those days, and at its conclusion Armstrong was received into the business house of the Openshaws, who were friends of the family, in Manchester. At the end of a year, however, one of the partners, who was himself a man of cultured tastes, and was interested in his young friend, realised that Armstrong was not of the material which makes the successful business man, and advised him to follow the strong bent of his inherent taste for art. He emphasised this advice by the practical action of a gift of money wherewith to make a start, suggesting Paris as the place for study. The serious adoption of an art career was looked upon somewhat askance at this time, especially in a prosperous community like Manchester, owing its well-being to trade, and it was only after combating family opposition that the definite step was taken, and he went to Paris in 1853, when he was twenty-one.

Though the date cannot be quite fixed, it is known that he studied at an art school in Manchester, where he and his friend John Thomson were regarded as unusually serious students. Very probably it was both before and after his stay in Paris.

He went there in June, and took a lodging first in the Rue Dauphine, and later in the Rue Fontaine, and in July entered the atelier of Gabriel Navier, in the Rue Chaptal, where he became a pupil of Ary Scheffer. Armstrong writes :—

I was furnished with a letter from Mr. Salis Schwabe to Ary Scheffer, at that time one of the most popular artists, with a European reputation. When I presented my letter I was set to work in one of the ateliers, and I used to draw from casts, and copy drawings and paintings, when there was no model sitting. I was deplorably inexperienced and ignorant, though I believed I knew a great deal. I have often thought how different my achievement might have been if I had been kept steadily to drudgery under the iron rule of such a master as Picot, the painter of the dullest and least interesting pictures of his time, but who knew what could be taught, and made his pupils follow his instructions. It is interesting to look through the old catalogues of the Salon fifty or sixty years ago, in which the names of the masters under whom the exhibitors studied are given, for most of the successful painters of that day had been trained under Picot, Heim, and Drolling, members of the Academy, but the most "stodgy" of all painters living. Decamps, for instance, was in Drolling's atelier, and he was an inventor and a colourist. When Scheffer came to see our work and direct us, we all stood until we were told to be seated. I think this was the practice too in other ateliers under the direction of famous painters. In this case the professor did not get any payment. The atelier was that of a favourite pupil who received the monthly fee, which in my case was twenty-five francs, and after paying the cost of models he kept the balance. In most of the large ateliers at that time one of the senior and most trustworthy students was made "massier," a kind of prefect, and managed the financial business in the professor's interest.

Socially Scheffer held a very important position, and had a detached house in a garden in the Rue Chaptal, with a large studio on each side of the avenue leading to it. One of these was a real atelier, or workshop, in which Legros and another paid pupil called Schotend used to work. Scheffer designed his portraits, and painted the heads and hands, and the rest was done by Legros, who copied his master's manner, and Scheffer worked thinly over the whole. The other atelier was beautifully furnished, and was very spick and span, with interesting works of art on the walls, and something very like a little chapel, in which were some works by the Princess Marie of Orleans, who had been a pupil of Scheffer's, or worked under him, until the time of her death. He was on very friendly terms with most of the sons of Louis Philippe.

In this grander studio musical parties were given, in which the most famous singers and instrumentalists of the day used to take part, just such as Leighton used to give when his friend Joachim was in London. I was never invited to either, and indeed one's professor was a long way off and above. The atelier in which I worked was on the opposite side of the street.

Armstrong studied in the evenings at Suisse's Academy, of which an account is given in the Paris reminiscences which follow in the second part of this volume.

The following notes regarding this time were written later.

The French artists I lived among, mostly in the student stage, knew little or nothing, even by hearsay, of British art; indeed they would ask "Est-ce que l'on fait de la peinture en Angleterre?" Some of them had heard of Hogarth perhaps and knew Flaxman's outlines, which were much esteemed. Bonnington's position was high, and a very large sum, considering market prices in those days, had been given for his little painting of François I. and his sister for the Louvre; but then Bonnington was looked upon as almost a French artist, and was personally well known in Paris.

There was a print shop on the Boulevard, not Goupil's, almost opposite the Maison Dorée, which generally had in its windows the excellent engravings after Sir Edwin Landseer's pictures, and these were much admired. But the favourable impression of the painter created by them was much diminished when some of his paintings were seen in the first International Exhibition of 1855, and it was then felt that Landseer owed a great deal of his reputation to the skill of the engraver. I remember that the painting of some of the early work of Ansdell was referred to as that of Landseer.

On the opening day of the Exhibition I saw a group of men, evidently artists, gathered round Mr. Holman Hunt's picture of *Strayed Sheep*, and I went behind them to hear if possible what they had to say about a kind of work so utterly new and unknown in Paris. I expected gibes, but in the short time my eavesdroppnig could be prolonged I heard the principal spokesman of the party say, " C'est étonnant comme cet homme a compris le caractère moutonnier." A very shrewd observation, for the sheep are huddled together in a way characteristically sheepish. This showed a disposition to recognise good qualities in work which in the main had no charm for the French painter of that day.

I tried to give Delacroix some idea of the pre-Raphaelite movement in England before the 1855 Exhibition was held, but I am afraid my attempt was a very lame one, for it is little use to try to give a correct impression of painting by words only. Delacroix had told me how he and Horace Vernet had been in London (I think it was in the thirties, and at the time when Géricault was in England), and how much they admired the work of the English painters of the beginning of the century, and of course the earlier masters, Gainsborough, Reynolds, and the rest. Constable was the English painter best known and most appreciated in France, and his pictures sent there for exhibition were much more relished and better understood than his work had been when shown in England up to that time. The Paris success re-acted in England, and counted for much in the recognition which came to him soon afterwards. Constable was looked on as the father of modern French landscape art.

After the Paris Exhibition more English students went to work in Paris, and there was a much wider knowledge here of modern French art. Until then Delaroche was the only French painter thought much of except Ary Scheffer, who was made popular chiefly through the engravings of his works, and neither of these painters was held of much account by the better sort of French artists. Later Rosa Bonheur achieved English popularity, and Edouard Frère jumped into vogue through Ruskin's praise of him in the press. He was a good painter, but his work fell off very much after he came to depend upon the English market.

Turner was unknown except by engravings, and not much even in that way. I believe there is some account in one of Delacroix's published diaries of my telling him about Turner's will, and the large fortune he left behind him. The accumulation of such a vast estate by painting seemed incomprehensible to the French artist.

The same lodgings were occupied for a year, when he moved into the Rue Chaptal under the ægis of the same landlady, until he was driven from it by "filth and vermin," and took refuge in the Hôtel Corneille, which was afterwards to contain so many associations for him. He joined forces there for a short time with a student named Cohen, from Savannah, and when he left for New York Armstrong remained there in a single room. In June, 1855, Paris was quitted for Antwerp, where he worked in the Royal Academy, but only for a couple of months, when he returned home. He stayed in England for a year, working in a room in his father's house in Manchester capable of being used as a studio, and in 1856 was again in Paris. His life, friends, and work there are later most graphically described in his own words.

In 1858, when he was twenty-six, he went to Algiers with his uncle, the Rev. William Evans, D.D., the only brother of his mother and the Staleybank aunts, who was seeking a mild winter climate. His aunt and two girl cousins were of the party. Armstrong bore an introduction from Alfred Elmore, R.A., to his brother, who was Vice-Consul at Algiers, Mr. Bell being the Consul. His knowledge of French and his geniality made him a great favourite in society. General MacMahon was the Governor at that time, and there were brilliant gatherings and balls at Le Palais, as Government House was called.

As recently as January, 1910, he refers in a letter to this visit:

It was the autumn of the great comet, and the spring of Magenta and Solferino. The colony of English and other foreigners was numerous,

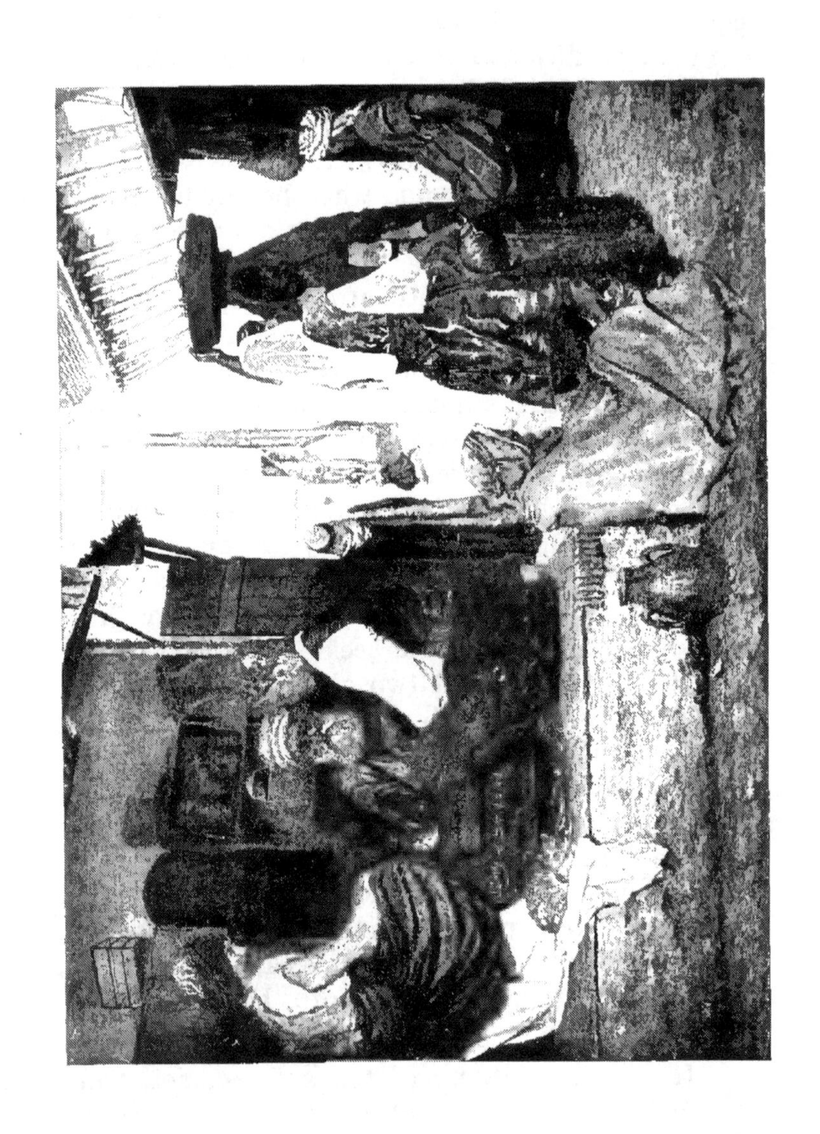

all known to each other, and there was much entertainment all through the winter. My relatives lived at the Hôtel d'Orient, I lodged all the time in a Moorish house kept by French people, close to the great Mosque, and had a studio in what was then the Rue Napoléon. At that time the difficulties of getting the natives to sit were almost overpowering. I was fortunate enough to sell all the pictures I did. It was a very happy time for me, and everybody was very kind.

He kept up a correspondence till his death, with Mme. Chassériaux, who had been Miss Bell, the Consul's daughter.

Armstrong writes, also in later years, of one of his experiences :—

There was a feast at Mustapha Inférieure on the coming into blossom of the bean, at which there was a very strange ceremony, and crowds of people came out of the town to take part in it. We were not early enough to see the sacrifice of an ox or a bull, which was the most important part of the proceedings. This was described to me by those who were earlier on the ground. When the beast was slaughtered the carcase was cut open, and a man, probably a negro, got inside it, and coming out covered with blood ran down the hill and into the sea. I regret very much not having paid more attention to this strange rite, for I was not so much interested in what now appears to me to have been a survival of the rites of the Taurobolium in the worship of Mithra as I was in the Moorish women, who were in tents guarded by negroes or older Arab women.

His relatives left in the spring, but he remained, extending his visit altogether to ten months.

In 1859–60 he spent some time in Düsseldorf, where du Maurier was also working, but unfortunately no details of his life there can be traced. The long friendship with John Chandler Bancroft, son of the historian of the United States, dated, for both du Maurier and himself, from this stay.

On his return to Manchester he continued his work at home, but presumably he was somewhat discouraged by lack of congenial surroundings, and felt himself at a standstill. Through his acquaintances the Renshaws, however, he was introduced to Mr. Jonathan Tong, which was the beginning of a lifelong friendship, and one that very considerably influenced his career. Armstrong gave Mr. Tong introductions in London to du Maurier, who was recently married, and also to Poynter and Marks ; and on his return Mr. Tong invited the young artist to his house to dine and to see his wife, as he had so thoroughly enjoyed meeting his painter friends in London. Mrs. Tong (now Mrs. Coltart) gives the following account in a recent letter :—

From the beginning to the end of the evening he was simply charming. When Mr. Tong returned from speeding the parting guest I said "Well ? " with a significant look. He replied, "Well, I feel as if I had never seen him before." Armstrong had evidently enjoyed his evening very much, and was in unusual spirits as he found himself in congenial society. He said he would like to show me photographs of pictures he had painted, so I fixed a day and he came and stayed two hours, talking most delightfully about art, and from that day onwards was our intimate friend.

An introduction was effected to Mr. William Coltart, who became the purchaser of a picture, on the proceeds of which a trip to London was made.

Not long after this he definitely left Manchester, to which he never returned to live, though he often visited his family, for he was a most devoted son He also frequently went north on professional matters.

He took rooms first in Great Russell Street, where he was close to the du Mauriers, who lived at number 91, and to whose little daughter he had stood godfather early in the year 1864. Life in town meant reunion of the Paris "gang"—Poynter, Lamont, Whistler, and du Maurier—as well as the formation of many new friendships. Mr. and Mrs. Burne-Jones were neighbours at number 62, and making their acquaintance led to the meeting of William Morris, T. L. Cobden-Sanderson, George Howard (afterwards ninth Earl of Carlisle), and William Nesfield, the architect. The firm of Morris, Marshall, Faulkner and Co. had been established in 1861, and its development was a source of constant interest. The decorative work, in which Armstrong was considerably engaged in the following years, brought him much in contact with Morris especially.

In August, 1864, he joined the du Mauriers at Whitby, their first visit of many, and while there he writes :—

I painted a picture out of doors, in the back garden, of children sailing a toy-boat in the harbour. This was long before there was any talk of plein air, which I think I first heard of from Fantin-Latour and the painters represented in his large group, Manet, Legros, Whistler, and others. . . . Croquet had just come into vogue, and we were all most enthusiastic about it. We played with the daughters of Dr. (later Sir) William Smith (distinguished by us as Dictionary Smith). Alfred Elmore, Henry (afterwards Sir Henry) Thompson, and Shirley Brooks, through whom I got to know the Leeches, were all staying in Whitby. When most of these visitors had left I began to see more of the Leeches. I walked with John every evening at dusk, and sometimes when the cliff was steep I had to give him an arm, for he was very weak, though we little knew how weak. Sometimes I went to see him by daylight, and found him always at work, for he was much driven, and day after day, when the usual number of blocks for Punch were done, he struggled with a kind of work he detested, and which he felt was of no artistic value. People used to say at the time that Leech lived extravagantly, but it was in consequence of his being called on by his family for help that he had to work all day during what should have been a health-giving holiday, and this work was of a heart-breaking kind. Most people have forgotten the enlarged versions of his sporting cuts, printed in colours, which were to be seen forty years ago in billiard-rooms all over the country. Some of these enlargements were made by a process of which the details are not known to me, and some were painted in oil colour on canvas by Leech himself, the outlines having been printed on them. He was not familiar with the use of oils, and the light-handed and sketchy manner by which alone, if at all, such painting could have been made attractive was not to be acquired off-hand. He told me that Millais, who was very much attached to him and would have spared no pains to help him in his difficulties, had shown him how it could be done. But without Millais's extraordinary skill with a paint-brush it was of little use to poor Leech, and it was strange Millais did not realise that.

It was only a few months later, early in November, that Leech died, and these extracts from two letters written by du Maurier to Armstrong, who was at the time in Manchester, serve to show the lovable attraction of Leech's disposition.

Like yourself, I had conceived quite a peculiar affection for Leech. He was so nice and kind on Friday, as indeed he always was, the dear fellow.

Keene came yesterday; he had heard the news on Saturday night at Lewis's, where Millais came in quite frantic it appears, just after Leech's death....He is to be buried on Friday at Kensal Green, next to Thackeray. Millais has just had a cast taken of his face....He died of sheer worry of mind in family affairs. Millais seems to have been a great brick, and to have taken everything on his hands, though terribly cut up.

Enfin, mon cher, c'est diablement triste; so young, too, only forty-seven. The gods must have loved him dearly. The funeral was a very painful and distressing business. I was asked to join the Punch party, and we met at the Bedford. You never saw such an affecting sight as when they put him into his grave. Millais suddenly burst out crying convulsively, and several others sobbed out loud, while the parson (Hole, who wrote that *Tour in Ireland*) read in a trembling voice and could hardly help breaking down too. Poor old Mark Lemon, as well; really it was quite awful, and I was so demoralized that my nervous system is hardly steady yet.

Silver told me that his domestic worries had killed him; it appears his father preyed upon him in the most unscrupulous manner, and that poor Leech had had to meet bills to the amount of £3,000 within the last two years....I saw the old fellow at the funeral, and recognised him by the likeness; the only dry eyes there.

The same peculiar fascination he had for us seems to have been quite general; everybody who knew him seems to have liked him, or rather loved him to a most extraordinary extent. You could see that yesterday. I have got to feel very warmly towards Millais through the whole of this sad business. There's no mistaking the deep and genuine affection he had for Leech.

Life in London was resumed, and the names which appear in his diaries—mere records of his daily work and engagements, severely without comments—represent all that was vital and of moment in the art community of the time.

Poynter had known Leighton in Rome, and

had sounded the praise of his various accomplishments, and he now, with Val Prinsep, became known to them all. Simeon Solomon was producing his highly imaginative work, and Charles Keene was busy over his inimitable black and white. He was a few years senior to Armstrong and du Maurier, having been born in 1823. After a five years' apprenticeship to Whymper, the engraver, he began to work on periodicals, and his association with Punch dated from about 1851. His long career with that paper, ending only with his death in 1891, lent the brilliance of a consummate artist to its pages. He was modest and reticent, but in a congenial environment and with his cherished pipe his charm of disposition manifested itself. Armstrong wrote about "bad language" being less common at the present time than when he was a young man, but also instanced people who were relieved by very simple expletives, and quoted Charles Keene, when vexed to extremity, saying: "I was so angry with him I could have said 'confound you!'"

The three Moore brothers, John, Henry, and Albert, formed a talented group, the first and the last of whom were on terms of the greatest intimacy with Armstrong and Lamont especially. The record of distinguished work in portraiture left by John Moore deserves wider recognition than it has ever received.

George Aitchison, architect, afterwards Professor and R.A., was a constant friend till his death in 1910, and he and Armstrong were collaborators in more than one decorative scheme. The most important of these was the dining-room at 52, Prince's Gate, carried out for the late Eustace Smith, M.P. The walls were gilded after a slightly indented pattern had been impressed upon them, an entirely new departure, which was acknowledged to be a most successful background for both people and pictures. The frieze was designed by Leighton, and the dado consisted of panels with inlaid designs of ivory, ebony, and mother-of-pearl. The two large pictures let into this wall were painted by Armstrong, and combined the most delicate effects of colour with strength of rendering.

A note which Armstrong wrote much later reads :—

George Mason and Aitchison were intimate friends in Rome, and the former used to speak of the bad times they had together there, when for a while they had neither money nor credit, and had to live entirely on polenta—a sort of porridge made of Indian corn meal. Aitchison was very sorry for himself, and said so one day when they were sitting grumbling together, but Mason reproved him, saying : "Oh ! well, this isn't very pleasant, but after all we have food of a sort, and you don't know how bad real hunger makes one feel." Then Mason went on to tell how after the misfortunes of his family, when his allowance from home came to an end and his credit was exhausted, and his spare clothes and trinkets had been parted with, and all the people he knew had left Rome for the summer, he fell into the direst want, and went for more than thirty hours with-

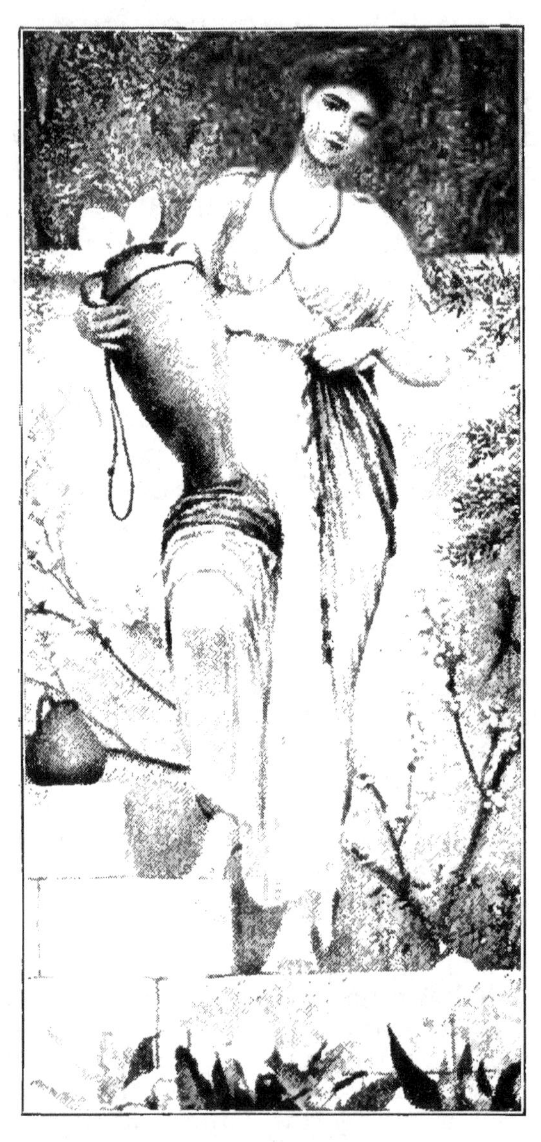

One of the two Decorative Pictures painted for the late Mr. Eustace Smith's Dining Room at Prince's Gate

out food of any kind. At this critical point he happened to remember that the children who went with their nurses to play on the Pincian Hill nearly always left bits of bread or buns about there, and so he went in search of some of these leavings. Having found a piece of bread he made off with it, and, hidden behind a tree, he tried to eat it, but he was nearly choked, and had the greatest difficulty in getting it down. In a lecture delivered at Hanley, Mason's native place, many years ago, Aitchison told this story, which caused no great surprise to those of Mason's friends who knew of the hard times he had gone through in Rome. Giovanni Costa, who knew most about Mason at this time, used to say there would never have been such a painter as Mason became if this pressure of poverty had not acted as a spur to effort.

Fred Walker (who was just about this time elected to the Old Water Colour Society), Marks, and Madox-Brown are among the many names of Armstrong's acquaintances.

A note from Burne-Jones, dated August, 1864, thanks Armstrong for the material benefit in "the promptest of cheques," of an introduction to Mr. Tong, he and his wife being most liberal patrons of his work, and also of that of other rising artists.

This is an early instance of what was throughout Armstrong's life so marked and lovable a characteristic—his untiring and willing service on behalf of his friends. No effort was spared, nothing was a trouble where a comrade could be helped, he had a genius for friendship. The response which his devotion called forth manifests itself in the fact that the intimate companionships of these early years held firm till the end.

Several houses were hospitably open to entertain these young painters. Armstrong himself tells of the family of the Ionides, with its several ramifications. Mr. and Mrs. Edwin Edwards surrounded themselves at their house at Sunbury with both English and French artists. Armstrong writes :—

I met Fantin for the first time while we were both guests at the house of Edwin Edwards, and found him most interesting in the exposition of his theories about painting as well as in his practice. While there he did a little still life painting of a highly coloured meerschaum pipe resting on the reflecting surface of a highly polished mahogany bookcase. There was much of unforeseen effect from these reflections, and on this account it was interesting and useful as practice, for no formula one had made would apply, and therein lies the use of studies of this kind, which force the painter to observe and see what the appearance or aspect really is, instead of being guided by what he thinks it ought to be.

Mr. J. P. Heseltine was in the happy position of being not only host but patron, and Mr. Arthur Lewis was famous for his entertainments, as a bachelor in Jermyn Street as well as after his marriage to Miss Kate Terry, at Moray Lodge, Campden Hill. Armstrong writes both from his own experiences and from those of du Maurier, which antedated his :—

Arthur Lewis was one of the foremost organisers of a body of part-singers, known first as the Jermyn Street Band, and later as the Moray Minstrels. Charles Keene was one of the most enthusiastic and regular attendants at the band, and most of the others were artists of one kind or another, Arthur Lewis himself being a good amateur painter, who had pictures in the Academy exhibitions. They were trained and led by Mr. John Foster, an alto, one of the Gentlemen of the Chapel Royal, more familiarly known among his friends as Johnnie Foster, who was a great favourite. After Mr Lewis removed from his rooms in Jermyn Street to the more spacious and sumptuous quarters at Moray Lodge these gatherings became less frequent, taking place only four times a year, but with a very numerous attendance. They had a great vogue, and people of all ranks sought for invitations, and no wonder, for the entertainment was of the most agreeable kind. The cards of invitation were designed by Fred Walker.

First came a set programme of glees and part-songs performed by the Moray Minstrels, and when that was over a good supper was served, in which oysters were an important feature. After supper volunteers were invited to amuse the company. Marks used to sing his comic songs and preach his American sermon, while du Maurier was always called on for some of his songs, by that time well known. I think that some of Gordigiani's were in highest favour (Gordigiani was Englished into Gaudy Johnnie), but *Le Vin à Quatre Sous* was always in demand.

Among the notable guests at these parties Millais was conspicuous from his stature and his handsome head, and his brother William's presence was also much prized on account of his beautiful tenor voice. William was rather short in stature and dark in complexion, but when you saw the two brothers side by side you were struck by many points of resemblance in their faces. I should never have guessed that Sir John had any Jewish ancestor, but he told du Maurier that he had, and was proud of it. On the other hand, in his brother William I should have recognised the Eastern type at once. The brothers' admiration of one another was amusing and sometimes touching. "Have you ever heard my brother Bill sing? He is the finest tenor you ever heard," Sir John would say; "his voice is far finer than Giuglini's." Giuglini was the great tenor opera-singer of the day. At the time of sending in the pictures to the Royal Academy, William would go about saying, "Have you seen Jack's pictures this year? Finest things ever done."

At Moray Lodge these gatherings became very large, and had perhaps lost something of their very friendly and intimate character when I first went to one of them and saw the early attempt at a theatrical performance. It was Offenbach's *Deux Aveugles*, given with du Maurier and Harold Power in the principal parts, and it was so successful that it was followed next winter by *Les Deux Gilles*, an operetta by a Belgian composer, and this again led to the composition of *Cox and Box*, a musical version of Morton's *Box and Cox*, with original music by Arthur Sullivan and new words by Burnand. In this piece Harold Power and du Maurier were again the principal performers, with Johnnie Foster or Arthur Cecil in the part of Sergeant Bouncer. I believe the first performance of *Cox and Box* was given at Sir Francis Burnand's house, and it was the second I saw at Moray Lodge; it was afterwards given more than once before a public audience, notably at Manchester, when the Punch authors and artists gave a representation in aid of a fund for the family of the artist, C. H. Bennett. I cannot remember how long afterwards *Trial by Jury*, with words by Gilbert and music by Sullivan, was produced at the Royalty Theatre; but it would appear that the genesis of the very notable series of operas, quite different from any imported works, and so charming, tuneful, and witty, that after their production an Englishman could look a Frenchman in the face, is to be found in the amateur performances at Moray Lodge, where Arthur Sullivan was a constant guest.

Armstrong tells in his own words how he made the acquaintance of Charles Reade in Paris, and he met him from time to time in London.

I first met Reade when I was copying Rosa Bonheur's famous picture of oxen ploughing, in the Luxembourg Gallery. This was in 1856, I think. He stopped to look at my copy, which I make bold to say was a very good one, and got into conversation with me and gave me his card. From what he said I gathered that he was an author of some note; but I had never heard of him, though *It's Never too Late to Mend* had been published some time and was most popular. I felt rather ashamed at having to confess that I knew nothing of his writings. Nothing much came of this acquaintance then, but long afterwards when I was in London I saw more of him.

He was a strange fellow; and another old friend of mine, Dr. Wheatley, who joined in rooms with him at Newhaven, near Edinburgh, about the time he wrote *Christie Johnstone*, said their landlady used to call him " Cracky Reade."

When I see the published portraits of celebrated or notorious persons lining the streets on big posters, or in the photograph shops, I often think of him and the answer he made when I asked if there were any published photographs of him to be bought. " Oh, dear no," he said, " and I'll take good care that there are none. Do you think my books would be bought and read with interest if people, especially in America, where my works sell best, knew they were written by such an unromantic-looking, chubby, and apple-faced fellow as I am ? " This was before he grew a beard.

There was hanging over the mantelpiece of the dining-room in his house in Bolton Row Millais' picture of *Sir Isambras*, and very splendid it looked there. Reade used to let this house for the season, and he told me that an old Scotch Countess came to look at it and seemed disposed to be his tenant, but she objected to the picture. She said, " I could not live in comfort in a house where such a picture as that would always be staring me in the face, with a horse twice the natural size." He told her he could not remove the picture, that she could not have the house unless she agreed to its remaining where it was, and showed her out ! This seems incredible, but I am convinced that he told nothing but the truth.

Many people have forgotten, if they ever knew, that Millais painted *Sir Isambras* in Perthshire, where there were no artists to come and see his work in progress and administer wholesome and corrective home truths, and he made the horse much too big for the man, too big even to represent the great, massive Flemish destrier which could bear the weight of its rider's armour as well as its own. The picture came to London to go to the Academy, and all Millais' friends were amazed when they saw what a mistake he had made—such a mistake as would have been impossible in London, where criticising artists would have come frequently to his studio. There was no time to repaint the horse, so Tom Taylor thought he would mend matters by providing for the catalogue some verses, purporting to be of the period, in which the gigantic bulk of Sir Isambras' charger was described. The artists, and for the most part the public, made fun of the big horse, and but few in those days recognised the great beauties of the rest of the picture. After the exhibition was over, the horse was repainted, and from an animal not at all like a heavy charger equal to fourteen stone of armour, not to speak of a man's body inside it.

Well, the point of my little story lies in the fact that the Scotch lady's objection was made to the size of the charger after this repainting was done! She had read in the newspapers that the horse was absurdly big, and that reached her *understanding*, the *sight* of the picture had no effect on her.

Sunday gatherings were frequent at Kew at the house of Mr. and Mrs. Courtenay Bell (she is sister to Sir Edward Poynter), of which pleasant recollections were always retained.

The friendship with Mr. Henry Wallis dates from the sixties. To the public he is familiar as the painter of *The Death of Chatterton*, now in the Tate Gallery, and to artists he is well known by his water colours as well as by his numerous volumes on ceramic art.

John Holker was, like Armstrong, a Lancashire man, and they first met in Manchester, where he was attached to the Northern Circuit. The friendship was renewed in London, whither he came in 1864, and always continued on a cordial footing. He rapidly stepped into a leading position, became M.P. for Preston in 1872, and was twice re-elected for the same constituency. He was appointed Solicitor-General in 1874 by Disraeli, with the usual knighthood, and soon after became Attorney-General. He returned to private practice at the end of Lord Beaconsfield's administration, and was enormously successful, performing many acts of unostentatious kindness to members of his profession.

Life settled down into something of a routine. The mornings were given almost unremittingly to work in the studio, more frequently from a model than not, though painstaking studies and experiments in methods were made for the pictures in progress. The work received criticism from brother artists, who with new friends in other professions came to the studio in the afternoons. He also received frequent visits from older friends who came to stay in town from the north. Dinner was the signal for a congenial gathering, as it fell into a custom for quite a large band of friends to meet at the same restaurant. In course of years the special house patronised underwent change, rising, as was to be expected, with the material progress of the patronisers. And naturally there were frequent changes in the men who formed the circle. In 1866 both Lamont and

Poynter married—Armstrong was best man to the latter—and their houses added to the number where evening or Sunday visits were paid. William Allingham was added to the circle of friends, and John Hare (then known privately as Johnny Fairs) is a name which constantly occurs in the diaries. London was flocking to see the Robertson plays at the Prince of Wales's Theatre in Tottenham Street, under the management of the Bancrofts, and Armstrong and his friends were loyal supporters.

There are many notes extant, making arrangements for meeting at both informal and formal dinners, followed either by visits to a theatre or concert, or only by the endlessly interesting discussions of their own and other people's work, present and past.

The following from Burne-Jones may be classed as informal :—

My deer armstrong

Som frends is a dinin here to morrow hevenin as is frens of yours mr and mrs howard and mr and mrs poynter, as is my sisterin law is dinin here and mr morris and mr stopford Brooke i didn no you was in town or else i would a ask you to do me the honour to jine and if the notis isn to short it would be a hegstream plesure if you was to jine its at harf past sevin polyticks is forbid because of divergen vews mr poynter and is good lady they been toris and mr morris rayther egstream contrariways and says mr howard isn as sound as he should be which makes the ground tickolish so we muss fall back on social scandle of which there is alwis plenty i do hope you will come as your cumpny is i mus say firs rate and me and my missus would take it kind if you was to come to dine tomorrow chewsdy at ½ pas 7 in the hevenin

i remain your offectionit

NED.

From 1865 onwards Armstrong exhibited in the Royal Academy, which till 1869 was still held in some of the rooms in the National Gallery.

In 1866 he spent the early part of the summer at Henley-on-Thames, lodging at a watchmaker's named Beck in the High Street, where there was a good garden at the back. To the same house also came Major and Mrs. Brine, just returned from India, with their two children, a maid, and a black Persian cat. The last-mentioned member of the party was the means of an introduction, for she was found one day eating Armstrong's evening chop, and the consequent apologies started a lifelong intimacy. The little girl, who fifteen years later became his wife, a particularly shy child, was nevertheless soon his fast friend, and when taken one day to be photographed entirely declined to be posed unless held closely by him.

His acquaintance with Madame Bodichon (Barbara Leigh Smith) added a very interesting personality to his circle. She was keenly in sympathy with all questions regarding the education of women, and was later one of the most generous benefactresses of Girton. When very young she had shown great artistic talent, and developed into a most accomplished painter, her

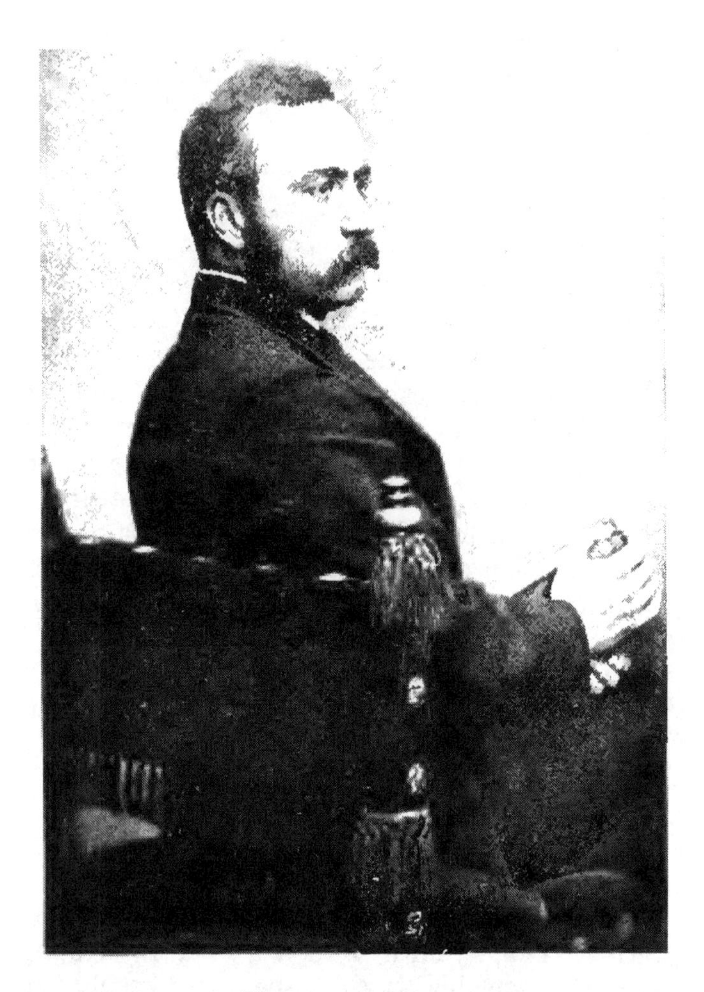

Thomas Armstrong
From a Photograph taken about 1866

gifts being recognised by William Bell Scott and D. G. Rossetti among others. She was intimate with Marian Evans, and was one of the very first to discover the identity of George Eliot, when the authorship of *Adam Bede* was still something of a mystery.

It was to her introduction that Armstrong owed his entry to the Sunday afternoon parties given at The Priory, St. John's Wood, of which he gives an account.

> It was considered a very great privilege to be allowed to attend these receptions, to which few but devotees were admitted; and it was not enough to be a devotee, one must also be in some way or other distinguished. I was a devotee, but I don't know how I came to appear distinguished enough to Madame Bodichon, who was an old and intimate friend of George Eliot's, and I felt as if I had been smuggled in under false pretences. I think I was more shy and awe-stricken the first time I was shown into the Presence at The Priory than I was the first time I went to Court. However, the great lady was very kind, and on my being introduced made me sit beside her on the sofa and talked to me very graciously until other guests arrived. I went again several times that summer, and was a good deal "set up" about having the entrée; but I don't think I really enjoyed the honour very much, for there was much solemnity about the gatherings, and one felt as if one must not speak above a whisper—at least I did. Smart people and people of rank, as such, had always been denied admittance, or, at least, had not been encouraged to come, and I only remember one

person of title among the frequenters. This was an old Irish countess, who was very pretty, and was always very well and fashionably dressed. Most of the ladies one met there, though intellectually much gifted and highly cultured, had a very serious, not to say dowdy appearance. I don't know how this sweetly pretty old lady came to be admitted, but I think she had been in the habit of coming for some time, though it appeared to me that she was regarded as an intruder, "a Levite without the gate," by the more serious of the devotees. She was very quiet and reserved, and did not assert herself at all.

Some time had passed without my going to offer my homage, when one Sunday afternoon I met a friend on her way to The Priory, and I turned back to accompany her. Most of the habitués were there, and others who came but seldom, so the gathering was more numerous than usual, and there was observable a remarkable vivacity among the male guests, which was uncommon. I found Lady C—— had brought with her a married daughter who had never been there before, and did not seem to recognise the sanctity of the place. She did not speak with bated breath like the rest, but talked freely and gaily to those about her, as she would have done in the drawing-room of a worldling. It was amazing for a new-comer to behave in this manner. The mother, who had been initiated long before, had never shown so free and easy a bearing in the sacred precincts. The daughter, Lady S——, was young, very pretty, and beautifully dressed, and it was interesting to see how her presence put the men on their mettle, and the talk became general and very lively. The conversation turned on Disraeli, and what was called his want of sincerity. Browning told us how, at the recent Royal Academy banquet, Disraeli in his speech had said that "However much the English school of painting might be defective in technical skill, it had at any rate that high imaginative quality which in art is beyond and above all others." Browning added that on a former occasion, at an Academy dinner, a speech had been made by Disraeli which contained a passage to the same effect. After the dinner, the speech-making being over and the guests strolling about in the galleries looking at the pictures as was the custom, the poet came upon the Prime Minister shuffling about with the gait those who have seen him must remember very well. Disraeli took Browning's arm, and walking along, with a glance now and then at the walls, exclaimed, "Tut, tut, not a single picture with the slightest trace of imagination in it." Someone suggested that Disraeli ought to have been reminded of this contradiction between his public utterance and his private conversation, but Browning had not then ventured on this step, and perhaps had not had the opportunity.

A friend who knew Mr. Gladstone very well told me later about the reception this story met with from him when Browning repeated it. "Yes, isn't it hellish ?" he said, "that's just the way he used to behave in the House of Commons." My friend could not see anything funny in it. I am sure that "hellish" was the word.

It was from Huxley that I heard long afterwards of Browning having found courage to remind Lord Beaconsfield of what he had said. The latter's comment was very characteristic: "My dear Mr. Browning," he said, "nobody but a poet would allow confusion to arise between what he says and what he thinks."

This story, which I admit is "tiré par les cheveux," has been told in print somewhere, but I am not aware that the last and most interesting part of it has been published. Lord Thring was so much delighted with Dizzy's apology that he made me give it to him in writing, but I don't know that he printed it.

Du Maurier became a favoured guest somewhat later. He was made much of, and used to sing for them, notably his little French song, *Fi de ces vins d'Espagne;* this became a general favourite at The Priory, where it seems to me the tone must have altered very much in a few years, and that this famous salon must have become "joliment dégourdi" to call for and relish so frivolous an entertainment. I wish I had kept up my visits and had been witness of the process of demoralisation.

Among the numerous original drawings in Mrs. du Maurier's possession there is a profile portrait done from memory of George Eliot, which I have been allowed to photograph. I have, however, never seen any drawing or portrait which gave a satisfactory impression of this distinguished lady.

In 1869 Armstrong moved to Charlotte Street, Fitzroy Square, where he lived for twelve years, occasionally hiring temporarily a second studio for the execution of some particular decoration or scheme of work. He was steadily gaining recognition as a painter, and very shortly after this time Sidney Colvin was writing of his work in The Portfolio, from which the following is quoted :—

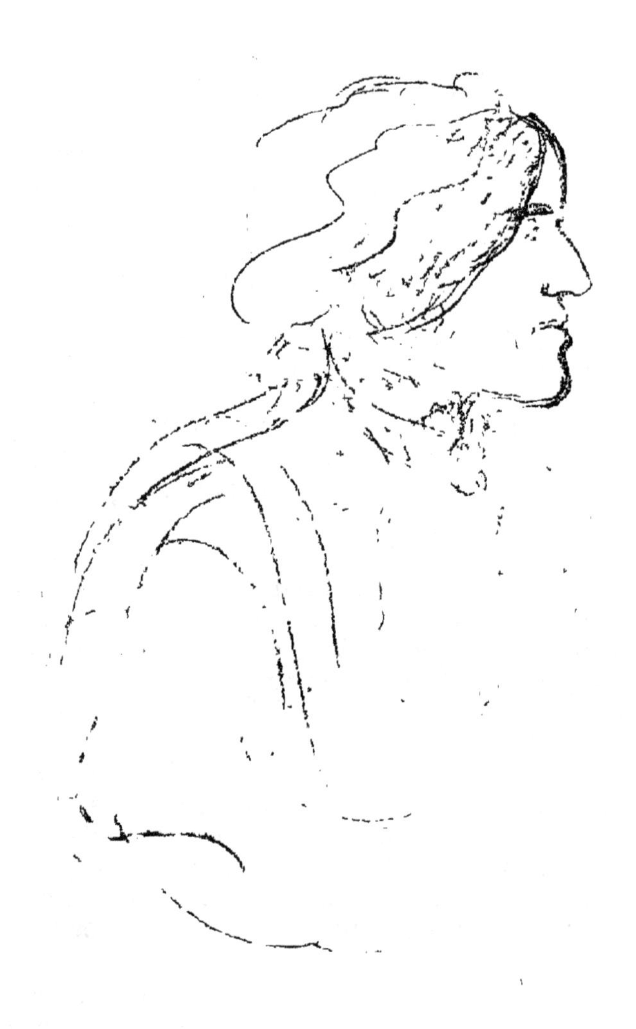

George Eliot
Pencil Sketch by du Maurier

There is a class of painters among us who, exhibiting year by year, never draw crowds or make sensations with their work, but nevertheless come insensibly to occupy positions of peculiar respect in the eyes of the more careful order of judges. To that class Armstrong belongs.... He has shown himself of those who see the raison d'être of a picture by no means in its subject interest, but altogether in its pictorial aspect and harmony. Whistler and Albert Moore are the two English contemporaries—both of them men of genius and breakers of new paths in our school—with whose work that of Armstrong is most in sympathy, though indeed he is as far as possible from being the follower of any individual leader. His modern range of decorative motives, as well as the quiet and almost Quakerly harmony of his favourite combinations in colour, are altogether personal to himself. What he does endeavour is to make every picture (that which in truth every picture ought to be) a careful and calculated object of pleasure for the eye in the arrangement of its forms and colours, neglecting at the same time no natural fact that he can manage, but choosing the subdued and delicate dealings of nature rather than those which thrust discords or brandish difficulties in the face of the spectator....For surroundings, for motive, for costume, Armstrong has been apt to turn towards the England of the eighteenth century, as who would not turn of such as care for simple refinement and reserve in outward things, for a natural and demure inventiveness in the accessories of life that is full of an inexpressible charm?

For some time Armstrong's Academy pictures were small in scale, but about two years ago there was a large picture on a system of mellow lilacs and greens, the result of very great care, with tall girls in a hayfield at sunset....the scene possessed by a delightful sense of summer, of evening, and of home. This year [1871], besides a very charming picture of a winter scene, there is a second, a still more satisfactory piece from the artistic point of view, an interior composition, full of delicate adjustments and very pleasant in colour, with two girls in easy chairs seated in profile in the foreground, and listening to the music of a priest who sits at his instrument in an inner room. In all these works it is just to say that purpose holds more place than power, and that the sedulous and guarded pursuit of admirable aims has not yet brought the artist beyond the stage subject to shortcomings, or put his work in possession of the look of ripe or plenary power and confidence. In the meantime, and at the stage where he is, his painting, with its conscientious care and balance, its tenderness and reserve, its aim at style and at pictorial charm, is of a kind on which the English school, more than another, has good reason to congratulate itself.

He made a separate study of one of the figures in the haymaking picture, which is mentioned above. It was bought by Lord Leighton, and hung always on the staircase in his house till the dispersal of his effects in 1896.

In all this time many Sunday evenings in each year were spent with the du Mauriers, who lived at Earl's Terrace, Kensington, after leaving Great Russell Street, before they migrated to Hampstead.

He saw a great deal of Edgar Barclay before he left England for Capri, and also of his friend

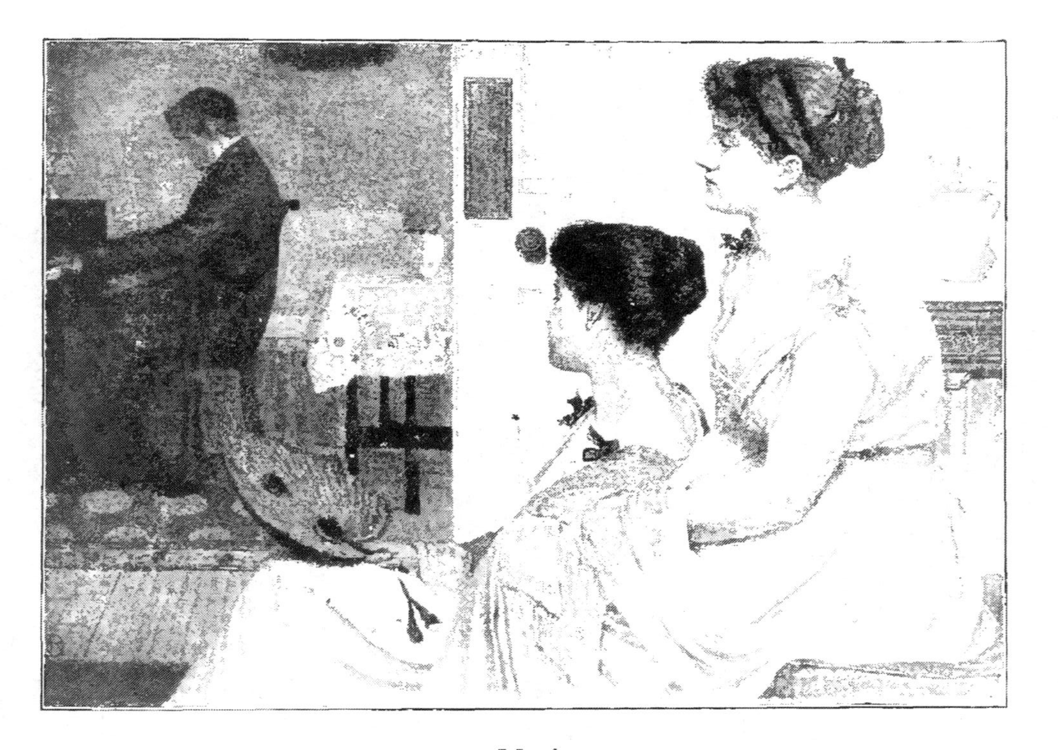

Music

Frederic Shields, who was in London at this time, though he had not yet definitely left the north. Sidney Colvin he met often, and he was always in touch with the men whose work was making the history of art, academic and progressive, in the last quarter of the nineteenth century.

In May, 1871, Randolph Caldecott came to London, the bearer of a letter of introduction to Armstrong, which proved the first link of a close and affectionate friendship, though it was not till twelve months later that Caldecott settled in town. They met, however, in the interim in Manchester, where Armstrong usually visited once or twice a year. Terms of the greatest friendliness and intimacy always obtained with Mr. and Mrs. Tong, who lived there, and he was constantly executing or superintending various decorative schemes with and for them.

He paid his first visit to Italy in 1872, accompanying Mr. Crook, a Manchester friend, on a tour of six weeks. He found time in a short halt in Paris to look up the Vinots, of *Trilby* celebrity, on the way to Milan. His brother Frederick lived there, so the travellers reaped the immense advantage, always appreciated, of being intelligently piloted about a strange city, and after a day spent at the Certosa of Pavia they went on to Verona, Padua, and Venice. A hurried visit was paid to Ravenna from Bologna, and then followed Florence and its environs, Siena, and Spezia. Sestri-Levante was reached by diligence, then train to Genoa. The Riviera was traversed to Marseilles, and after seeing Arles Armstrong and his friend returned to London by Paris and Boulogne. All this ground was later to become familiar, as this proved to be the first of numberless journeys to Italy.

He worked on a portrait group of the three elder children of George Howard on his return to London, and later in the year visited the family at Naworth Castle, where Leighton and Sir William Vernon Harcourt were also guests.

Armstrong and Caldecott met almost daily, and the dining circle at Greliche's, a restaurant just off Oxford Street, near Poland Street, comprised, besides Lamont, Mr. Joseph Wallis, architect, Albert Moore, Allingham, and occasionally Mr. Henry Blackburn, who became well known as the editor of *Academy Notes*, amongst many others. Dinners were now also frequent at the Arts and Savile Clubs, of both of which he was a member at this date.

The old acquaintance made in Paris, William O'Connor, was in London for a time, warmly welcomed by the "gang," and William Bell Scott, as well as Rossetti, Inchbold, Felix Moscheles, Frederick Burton (afterwards Director of the National Gallery), George Leslie, and Mr. and Mrs. Westlake, were friends of this period. W. B. Scott was both poet and painter, son of Robert Scott, the Scotch engraver. He began to write when very young, and sought advice from the great authority in Edinburgh circles, Christopher North. Scott came to London, and sent in a cartoon to the competition for the decoration of the Houses of Parliament. Though not successful it procured him an appointment to the Newcastle School of Design, a position he held for many years, and which carried with it the organisation of art education in the north. Among his chief paintings were elaborate decorations on Border subjects for Sir Walter Trevelyan, at Wallington Hall, Cambo, and a series of designs for Miss Alice Boyd, of Penkill Castle, a very intimate friend, illustrating the *King's Quhair*. When he and Rossetti were both guests at the Castle, and the latter had been throwing off some of his nonsense verses, it was said Scott sat up most of a night vainly endeavouring, in retort, to find a rhyme to Rossetti. He produced several volumes of poems containing work of some distinction.

J. W. Inchbold was a painter of pre-Raphaelite tendency, whose work, though delicate in feeling, failed in attraction on account of a certain hardness and coldness. He was an intimate member of the society in which Armstrong moved, and, like Armstrong himself, possessed the power of evoking and preserving warm friendships.

Early in 1873 he was again in Milan, summoned by his brother's illness. When there was no longer cause for anxiety and he was free to go out, he worked at designs in the Brera, and visited and noted details in the Ambrosian Library and the churches. In February he went by Savona to Mentone, where he sketched in the olive gardens and made landscape studies. He was drawn back by an unfailing attraction to paint again and again in this country. On his return to England he was engaged upon work which peculiarly fitted his tastes, in which he was associated with his friend W. E. Nesfield. The latter had received a commission from Mr. Henry Renshaw to remodel Bank Hall, near Chapel-en-le-Frith, Derbyshire, and Nesfield suggested the decorative panels for the dining-room should be entrusted to Armstrong. He, in his turn, collaborated with Randolph Caldecott, who painted all the birds, which formed a feature of the decoration. It was his first work in oils. One of the panels is reproduced. Before the work was fixed in its place it was exhibited at Deschamps' Gallery in New Bond Street, framed in its oak mouldings, and attracted much attention.

John Bancroft was in London this year, which was always the occasion of friendly meetings with Armstrong, du Maurier, and Whistler among others. A large London acquaintance had resulted from his father having three times filled the position of American Minister at the Court of St. James.

Mrs. Mark Pattison, a friend for whom he had warm admiration, sat to him, and also Mrs. Hennessy, the beautiful wife of his artist friend, W. J. Hennessy. Caldecott and Lamont he saw constantly, and Sundays were sometimes spent with friends on the river, or at Farnham Royal, where Mr. and Mrs. Henry Blackburn had a cottage.

Mr. F. B. Seaman, a great friend of Caldecott's, frequently made one of the chosen circle at the Progrès, which was the restaurant most in favour at this date.

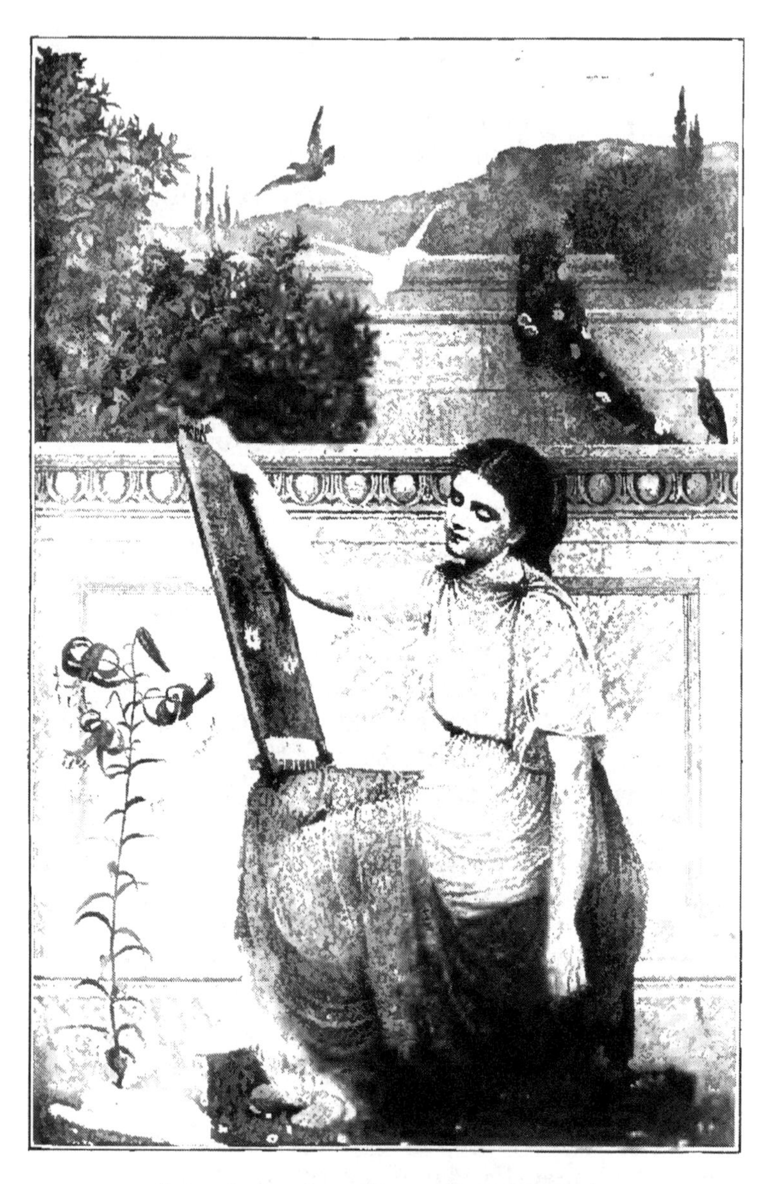

One of the three Decorative Pictures painted for the Dining Room at Bank Hall

An interesting visit was made to Cambridge in December, 1874, to hear Colvin lecture at the Fitzwilliam on Luca Signorelli, when he dined afterwards at Trinity with Henry Fawcett, Arthur Balfour, and Henry Sidgwick.

In 1875 he was much engaged for several months on the work at Broome Hall, Holmwood, the decoration of which was being carried out, under his supervision, for his friend Mr. Pennington, and he was constantly backwards and forwards there. Caldecott was again associated with him in this work.

In the autumn of this year Caldecott's illustrations to *Old Christmas* were produced, and at once made a mark, which was a source of pleasure to Armstrong, foremost among his friends.

The work at Broome Hall occupied some months of 1876 also. He paid his usual visits to Manchester, and used to meet old friends at the Brasenose Club there. Among them was William Percy, who painted portraits, both water-colours and miniatures. He had done an excellent picture of the aunts, the Misses Evans, of Staleybank, mentioned earlier, seated on either side of their parlour window, their faces and figures in profile, which gave a quaint and attractive effect. Percy was an early sympathiser with Armstrong's tastes, and helped him considerably in the start of his career, aid which was cordially repaid when misfortune befell Percy in later life. Besides his relations at Prescot, he always saw a great deal of his friends Mr. and Mrs. Tong at Breeze Hill, when staying at his father's house.

He was constantly dining out at one or other of his large circle of friends in town. Whistler he saw from time to time, and met George Meredith more than once, dining at Mr. Lionel Robinson's and elsewhere. He gave afternoon parties at his studio, where about this time he had great intercourse with Miss Gertrude Jekyll, the two Miss Townshends, and others, over embroideries for curtains, and various hangings. He took great trouble over the materials, designs, and colours, often making experiments in dyeing with his own hands. It must be remembered how large a debt is owed to the pioneers of this revival of the art of embroidery in the facility with which beautiful fabrics of varied and harmonious colourings can now be bought.

Miss Jekyll writes the following note, which she speaks of as a "poor tribute to a nearly life-long friendship."

During the time between (and including) the years 1871–1877 I often met Mr. Armstrong. Problems of colour and design as applied to needlework greatly interested me, and no doubt, owing to the influence of William Morris, it was becoming possible to obtain a better choice of coloured material to work upon and to work with.

Some needlework of mine had been in one of the international exhibitions, and had been seen by Leighton, who was then unknown to me. Greatly to my pride and gratification he had asked me through a common friend to do some embroidery for him. It was probably some of this that I first showed Mr. Armstrong. He had numbers of friends in the world of fine art, and through him many commissions for needlework

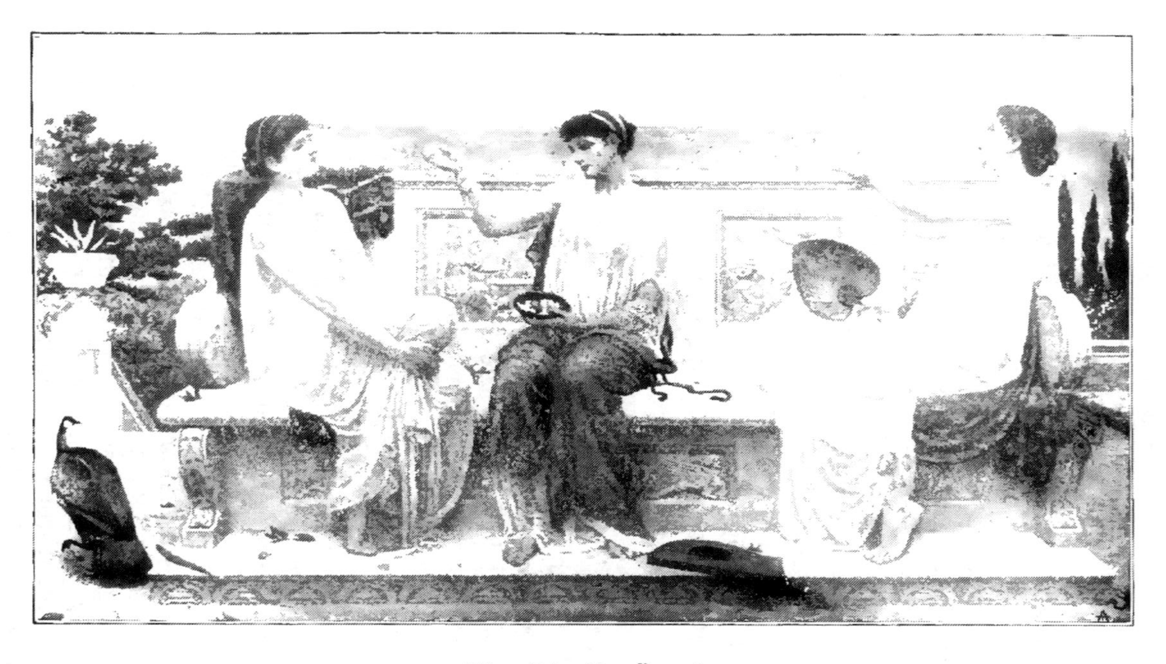

The Marble Bench
Now at South Lytchet Manor

came to me. I was conscious of learning much from his finely developed sense of colour, and was greatly cheered and encouraged by his always ready helpfulness and sympathy.

After Pinwell's death there was an exhibition of his work at Deschamps' Gallery, in February, 1876, which naturally excited much attention, mingled with regret that his fine talent and original sense of beauty should have ended at the early age of thirty-three.

Sir John Holker commissioned a picture and Armstrong painted *Feeding the Robin* for him; and Mr. S. Pope, Q.C., bought *Three Women on a Bench*, a picture which was very popular and often lent to exhibitions. It was sold at Christie's on Mr. Pope's death, and is now in the possession of Sir Thomas Lees, at South Lytchett.

He kept continually in touch with his immediate circle of friends, du Maurier, Poynter, Lamont, Caldecott, and Walter Crane, to whose son, Lionel, he was godfather, and met Spencer Stanhope at Burne-Jones's and elsewhere when he was in London; also Sanderson, who was tutor to Lady Amberley's sons. In the autumn he stayed at Shaldon, Teignmouth, sketching and boating, part of the time as guest to Colonel and Mrs. Brine.

Caldecott, after the production of his illustrated edition of *Bracebridge Hall*, a sequel to *Old Christmas*, went to Mentone, seeking health. The cordial terms of this comradeship were never interrupted, and the encouragement given by

Armstrong's heralding of his friend's charming and individual work was always appreciated. Armstrong joined him on the Riviera in February, 1877, where they sketched in the garden of the Hôtel Splendide and elsewhere, until Armstrong was recalled to Manchester on family affairs.

Sir Coutts Lindsay had been preparing for some time the scheme of his Grosvenor Gallery, and an enormous interest was felt in the art world at the launching of this new venture. It was thought the tactics were to be the ignoring of the Academy, as exhibition was by invitation only. But though the best work which did not find favour at Burlington House was included in this "very select exhibition," it appeared that Leighton, Millais, Poynter, and others had not been excluded. Armstrong was among those approached, and became a regular exhibitor from its earliest days till his appointment to South Kensington. He sent a seapiece he had worked on at Shaldon to the first exhibition.

Caldecott's delicacy, a source of constant anxiety to his friends, obliged him to give up all work for a time, and he was ordered to Shaldon for change of air in May. Though irked by the prescribed idleness he wrote, as was his manner, very amusing letters to his intimates. Those that he sent at different times to Armstrong are of so private a character that it is difficult even to make extracts from them. He said in a letter to their mutual friend, Henry Blackburn, in 1876: "Pen can never put down how much I owe in many ways to T. A."

His list of engagements shows how sedulously Armstrong was sought as a guest, but the mere recital of these dinners and parties forms but an arid record. They were interspersed with unremitting work and the usual meetings with his immediate circle, but there are no amplified accounts with which to clothe the bare facts.

Mr. William De Morgan and his sister are mentioned as fellow-guests at dinner with Burne-Jones at 1, Palace Green (Mr. George Howard's), an intercourse which, though already of some standing, was later to become more frequent. It was in this year that his old friend Leighton was chosen President of the Royal Academy, a position he filled with extraordinary distinction.

Armstrong was absent from London for some months, as he was staying in the north when his father was taken ill and died on June 16th. His mother survived him one week only, and passed away on the 22nd. They had both lived on into old age, and Armstrong was ever full of tenderness in his relation to his parents. He inherited many of his attractive qualities, especially his unselfishness, from his mother, a woman of a beautiful character. During her last years she had suffered from a painful and depressing disease of the eyes, and her son's constant thought for her, his visits and his frequent letters brought comfort to her in her saddened and inactive life.

In such a break in the home life there was naturally a great deal of family business to be settled, and he stayed on with his sister for some time.

He saw a good deal of George Howard, Spencer Stanhope, Burne-Jones, and Walter Crane on his return to town at the end of July. Caldecott, whom he saw constantly, had been in Brittany with Henry Blackburn, the outcome of which tour was *Breton Folk.* He was now very busy over his Picture-Books as well as on the Graphic and other work. His health, unhappily, made absence from England obligatory, and he left for the Riviera in late autumn.

In 1879, and for two or three years afterwards, Armstrong worked at intervals on a picture known as *The Flight into Egypt,* which was eventually bought by Mr. Westlake.

He had become a member of the Society for Preservation of Ancient Buildings, and attended its meetings, where he met several professional friends, George Aitcheson among them. The proposed restoration of St. Mark's was one of the points then under consideration.

In April he went to Mentone, and spent rather more than a month there, working from models and sketching from nature. He then visited his brother in Milan, and during his stay made himself intimate with the churches, libraries, and museums. An instance of Leighton's facility for languages is noted in the following account:

My brother took me to the house of the Countess Borromeo, where I met people interested in art. They were talking about a recent banquet given in the city in honour of Massareni, a senator, who was also known as a writer and

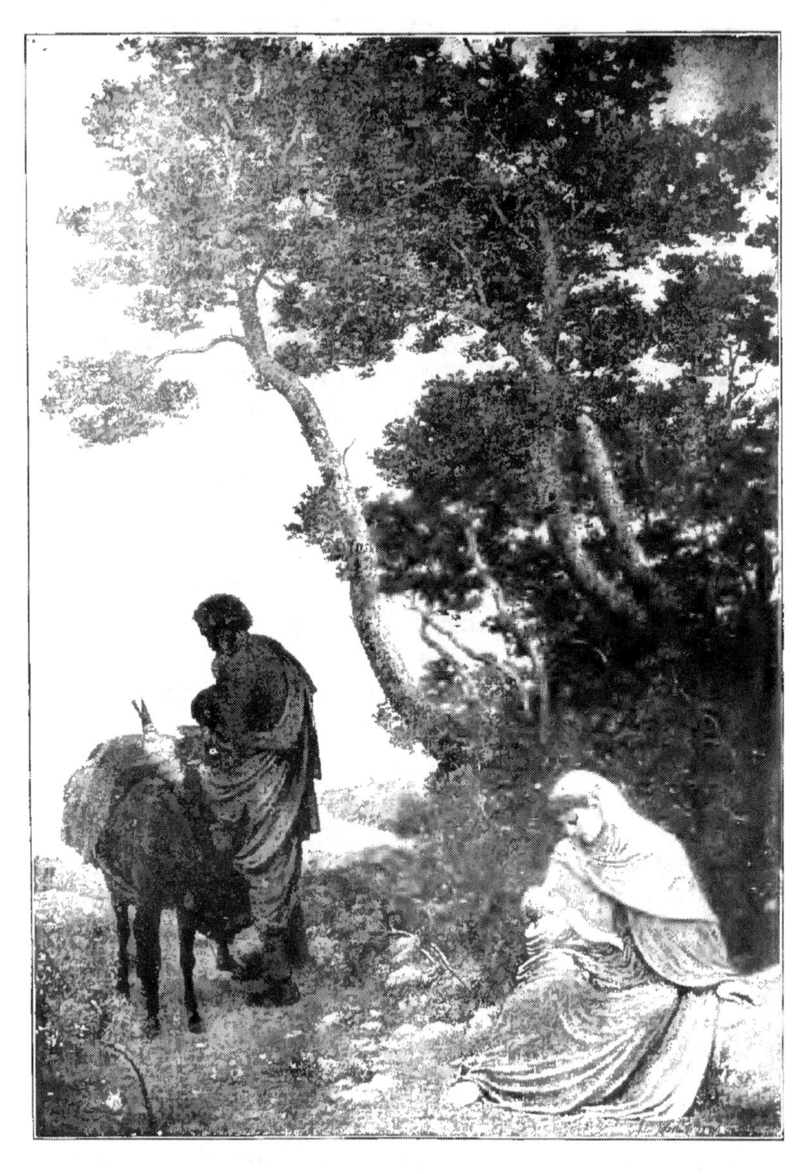

The Flight into Egypt
Now at The River House, Chelsea

art critic. On the morning of the day's "sollennité" some of the committee heard that Leighton was in Milan, and a member was deputed to go to his hotel and invite him to the dinner, to which he came. The toast of the evening was, of course, Massareni, to which he replied in an eloquent speech in Italian (at that time the Milanese, gentle and simple, among themselves spoke Milanese). Afterwards Leighton's health was proposed, and he in reply made a still more eloquent speech than Massareni's, in even more elegant and correct Italian.

Leighton used to go every year to Perugia, and in gold medal years at the Academy when he had to prepare an oration he stayed there a month, occupying the same rooms in Madame Brufani's hotel. A friend of Costa's, an artist of merit, Count Lemmo Rossi Scotti, lived a few miles out of Perugia at Sta. Petronella, and he was pressed to call and make the acquaintance of the President, who, as is well known, was a very warm and close friend of Giovanni Costa. Rossi Scotti, a very diffident man, told me how, after much persuasion, he went to the hotel and asked for Leighton, and waited for him to be fetched. By and by a handsome gentleman came in speaking perfect Italian with a very strong Tuscan accent, and addressed him. Rossi Scotti said, "I am sorry to have deranged you, but there is a mistake for I came to see an English gentleman."

On his return to town in July, 1879, he was busy seeing his friends. He met Giovanni Costa, with and at the George Howards', and there is mention of his being Armstrong's guest with Edgar Barclay and Spencer Stanhope at the Arts

Club. He went north in August, where there was still some family business to settle, and he also superintended the memorial erected to his parents in Birch churchyard, which was entirely of his own design.

As was always the case when they were both in London, he and Caldecott met constantly. This autumn the latter had taken a small house—Wybournes, Kemsing, near Sevenoaks—and Armstrong seems to have contributed some furniture for it. He helped him to settle in, paying other visits there also, which usually meant going to Chelsfield as well, where Miss Marian Brind lived, to whom Caldecott was engaged to be married.

The late autumn saw him again in Manchester, as his old home at Fallowfield was sold, and the business connected with it required his attention. In December he and his sister, Miss Armstrong, with other relatives, started for Mentone, where they took up quarters at the Hôtel Splendide, and Mr. Frederick Armstrong joined them there for Christmas.

The first six months of 1880 were spent abroad. He hired a studio at Mentone, and the pictures he had been working on in London were sent out to him there. Miss Armstrong fell ill, and was invalided for a time, but was gradually able to join in the excursions made in the neighbourhood. As in London, he worked usually in the mornings and he found suitable and pleasing models at hand. Society was not lacking, as there were friends and acquaintance at Mentone; among others James Bruyn Andrews, son-in-law of Cyrus Field, associated with the first Transatlantic cable. Their friends the William Oslers were at the Villa Claire. He kept up a large correspondence with London friends, and very often despatched flowers, a custom not so common then as now. He sketched a great deal on his walks, treasuring various effects in this country which made so strong an appeal to him.

In February they all went to Genoa, where he parted from his sister and the other members of the party, and returned to Mentone and his work while they journeyed on to Florence. He saw the Edward Greens, old north-country friends, who stayed for a time in Mentone, and spent his evenings usually with people he knew in the place. Excursions were made both to Ventimiglia and to Bordighera, where Armstrong had acquaintances.

He sent off pictures for the summer exhibition at the Grosvenor Gallery, and in May he left Mentone and joined his sister at Florence. His first visit had been brief, so there was a great deal new to him. He went constantly to Mr. Spencer Stanhope's villa at Bellosguardo, and was introduced to the circle of friends gathered there.

The homeward journey for them all began by travelling to Bologna on the way to Milan, where Armstrong acted as cicerone to the party, staying with his brother while the others were at an hotel; and early in June they all left for Paris, whence Armstrong returned to Charlotte Street by himself. Caldecott had married in March, so the bachelor ways and customs could not be resumed, but, as had been the case with Lamont and Poynter, the marriage had but further cemented the friendship.

In October he went on a round of visits—to the Edward Greens at Snettisham in Norfolk; to Mr. and Mrs. Tong at Breeze Hill, Manchester; to Naworth Castle, where Mr. Edward Hughes was also a guest, and where he painted with his host, George Howard, in his studio; to relatives in Newcastle, going back to Manchester before his return to Charlotte Street.

In December he went to Shaldon, Teignmouth, and did a good deal of work there, though his interest was not, just now, absorbed in his painting, his engagement to Miss Alice Brine following very shortly on this Devon visit.

MEMOIR
1881-1911

II.

1881–1911

The year 1881 brought great changes into Armstrong's life. In April he was married to Miss Brine at the British Embassy in Paris, and in the autumn his official career began upon his appointment to the Science and Art Department at South Kensington.

After the marriage he and his wife went to Mentone, where Mr. and Mrs. Caldecott were then staying—a visit of enjoyment in its present, and a source of happiness to remember in its past. A sudden move was made, as news reached them of the dangerous illness at Milan from typhoid of Armstrong's old friend Mr. Tong. Upon hearing of his death they went at once to Mrs. Tong, and, as they both so well knew how, rendered her every possible help in her trouble. The funeral took place on 8th May, and Mrs. Tong left the next day for England. After returning to Mentone, on a visit to their friends the Oslers, they travelled back to London.

In July Armstrong was first approached by George Howard in respect of the appointment at South Kensington, which involved succession to part of the work hitherto carried on by his old friend Sir E. J. Poynter, whose retirement was due to lack of leisure for his own painting. There were many interviews with Lord Spencer, Mr.

Mundella, Leighton, and others, and on 7th September Armstrong received the official offer of the post, which he wrote to accept on the 8th, and received the keys of office on the 22nd. October 3rd saw the official starting of his work as Director of the Art Division and Art Adviser of the Science and Art Department of the Committee of Council of Education.

On his acceptance of the post he received a cordial letter of welcome from Earl Spencer, who was then Lord President of the Committee of Council of Education. This was the beginning of an intercourse which grew to be most sympathetic, as numerous letters testify. Lord Spencer had absolute confidence in Armstrong's knowledge and judgment about pictures, old and new, and often consulted him about the treatment of those at Althorp.

At this time Mr. and Mrs. Armstrong had no settled home in London, and there was a proposal of combining with the Caldecotts, a house in Cheyne Walk being inspected to that end, but finally the scheme dropped. They were, however, just now brought a good deal in contact with Chelsea, as their friends Mr. and Mrs. Westlake were settling into a fresh house which had been built by Mr. G. F. Bodley, R.A., on the Embankment, and Armstrong's taste was largely consulted as regards its arrangement and decoration.

In December Armstrong made his first inspection of the Art Schools of Exeter, Bristol, and York, work with which he was shortly to become so familiar. Early in 1882 Mr. and Mrs. Armstrong moved into 14, Sheffield Gardens, Campden Hill, which was their home for the next eleven years. His work involved a good deal of travelling about, and in March he was in Dublin, of which visit he gives the following account, written many years after:—

The first time I went to Ireland on official business it was to try and bring to order the masters of the Metropolitan School of Art in Dublin, who had been for some time very rebellious and troublesome. My predecessor, Sir Edward Poynter, had been sent on a similar errand about two years earlier, but the effects of his chastening had not been lasting. I have nothing of importance to record about the school except that these troublesome masters were Englishmen, and when on returning I told Lord Spencer (who had sent me) that I thought an Englishman after being some time in Ireland was given to deteriorate: "Yes," he said, "that's what people said to *me* when I came home after being Lord Lieutenant."

He was so very kind as to write to Lady Cowper about my visit, for Lord Cowper was at that time Viceroy, and on the morning after my arrival there came to my hotel a dragoon with an invitation to dine at the Castle that same evening. The Irish porter was much impressed by this, and I felt that my social position was established, so I was much "set up."

I met their Excellencies at a picture exhibition during the morning and so made their acquaintance, and in the evening at the appointed time made my way to the Castle in a cab. I was shown into a small ante-room, where I found several men wearing the livery of the staff—a dress coat lined with light blue silk, which was retained on the lappels. Other men and some ladies soon joined us, but I was the only guest from outside. I think Mr. Forster, who had that day returned from making his defiant and courageous speech from a window at Tullamore, and Sir Thomas Steele, the Commander-in-Chief, lived in the Castle. Lord and Lady Cowper came in, there was a blare of trumpets, doors were thrown open and we marched into the dining-room, but I cannot remember in what order. We sat at a round table, the decorations on which were in good taste, and the room had a cheerful and sumptuous appearance. The dinner was excellent, and the conversation was friendly and lively. In the quadrangle below a band was playing, but the music was not unpleasantly loud, and was never a bar to conversation. At some signal which I did not perceive the trumpets blared again, and we rose for the ladies to leave the room, the ladies-in-waiting curtseying to the Lord Lieutenant before retiring. My next neighbour, his sister-in-law, made her obeisance with a sort of wink, which took away some of the solemnity; but the whole proceeding was very stately and impressed me much, for I have never before or since been present at so regal a function. The lunch Queen Victoria gave us in St. George's Hall, Windsor, when I and some thirty or forty others went to be invested, was on a larger scale, and from the fact of all the men being in uniform of some kind or other had a great show of colour, and moreover the Flaxman gold plate was on the table; but even so, it did not impress me so much as this Dublin Castle dinner.

In a report on a visit to Paris in May of this year he says that "he noted all the examples of which casts were obtainable." He was profoundly impressed by the support given by the state to art schools and education :—

> The state gives with a liberal hand and the municipalities seem to vie with it....In the schools pains and money are not spared to give students fresh sharp casts, kept clean, to draw from, and care is taken to place them in the best light, both by day and night. These are matters of the first importance. The Department would do well to procure specimens of some of the fittings we saw.

He established the most friendly relations with the foreigners whom he met, and his genial manner often overcame obstacles which in the hands of a less skilful diplomatist would have proved insurmountable.

The remainder of 1882 was largely taken up in travelling on the business of the Department. When in London he met George Howard constantly, as he used his studio in Palace Green whenever he could find time for private work. The official note of his appointment specified : " He will not be required to give his whole time, but will act as Inspector of the provincial schools of art. He will also advise as to purchases and general arrangements of the art branch of the Museum." But in practice it was found that each year made greater demands upon his time, and so a fresh arrangement was made which entailed the abandonment of his own work, and he devoted himself unreservedly to the service of others.

In April, 1883, the only child of the marriage was born, Ambrose George, his father's old friends George Howard, T. R. Lamont, and Mrs. Caldecott standing as sponsors.

The close intimacy with the Caldecotts was maintained, though naturally the change to official life brought many fresh personalities into the circle of friends and acquaintances. Among these were Sir John Donnelly, to whom he was already known, who was Secretary to the Science and Art Department, and Sir William Abney, who was then Assistant Director for Science, and later succeeded Donnelly as permanent head of the Department. Sir Philip Cunliffe Owen was Director of the Art Museum for several years after Armstrong's appointment, and was succeeded in the post by Dr. J. H. Middleton in 1893, who held it till 1896 only, when Sir C. Purdon Clarke filled his place.

Professor T. H. Huxley was Dean of the College of Science, and General E. R. Festing was first Assistant Director and later Director of the Science Museum. Mr. J. Hungerford Pollen was Assistant Keeper of the Museum, Member of the Committee of Selection, and official Editor to the Department. Mr. J. C. Sparkes was principal of the Training School (afterwards Royal College of Art). There were constant meetings, naturally, of these different servers of the Museum, and Armstrong's genial personality was a passport to friendship amongst them. The Green Dining-Room of the Museum took the place of Gréliche's and the Progrès of earlier days.

Of a visit to Rome in December, 1883, he writes :—

At this time Mr. (afterwards Sir George) Errington was in Rome, covertly representing the British Government at the Vatican, and my first step was to get into communication with him. It should be mentioned that Mr. Gladstone was badgered frequently in Parliament about the nature of Mr. Errington's mission, but in reply to questions he would never admit that he was acting officially as the agent of the British Government. Perhaps in doing so he framed his answers in such words as to leave a loophole for his conscience, but he certainly meant his words to convey the impression to his hearers and the public that Errington had no authority to negotiate with the Pope.

I saw Errington very frequently, and breakfasted with him, meeting at his table people from the Vatican. Among them was M. Henri des Houx, editor of the Pope's French newspaper. I was very much interested in his conversation, and was moved to say to him that he ought to publish his recollections. He replied that much of what he was saying could not be made public, and I suppose it was so. I remember the subjects of our conversations were mainly about obtaining the Pope's veto against the appointment of Archbishop Walsh. It was hoped in England that His Holiness might make this concession to our Government, and Errington's principal business in Rome just then was to obtain it. A possible equivalent for this favour was freely discussed. I remember des Houx saying: "It is a case of 'Do ut des,'" pointing out that the despatch of a British man-of-war to take an

Archbishop or Patriarch to or from Malta could hardly be counted as a sufficient return. Errington was quite sanguine about succeeding, but from what I heard I never believed that he could offer any substantial return; and it turned out that I was right. These people talked freely enough before me, just as if I had been a "papalino." My business in Rome with the Vatican was threefold: to get permission to have a cast made from the Venus of Cnidus; to get leave to make a model of one of the rooms of the Appartamento Borgia decorated by Pinturicchio; and to have copies made of the three pieces of tapestry designed by Raphael, of which the cartoons have disappeared. Four hundred pounds had been given for this purpose by a private person, an expenditure with which I personally did not warmly sympathize.

My chief interest was in the Appartamento Borgia, which was a revelation of beauty to me. At that time it was very little known, for the four rooms of which it consists were used as an annexe to the Vatican Library, where rare books and codices were stored. Monsignor Ceccolini, who for a long time had charge of the Library, was very jealous of intrusion into his domains, for he said the Library officials could not be held responsible for the safe keeping of the documents stored there if strangers were allowed to work in the rooms; and, indeed, he complained that valuable things had been taken away by some of the few visitors who had been admitted. This determined opposition to the scheme for making the model was very discouraging. I was told that nobody would ever be allowed to work long enough in the appartamento.

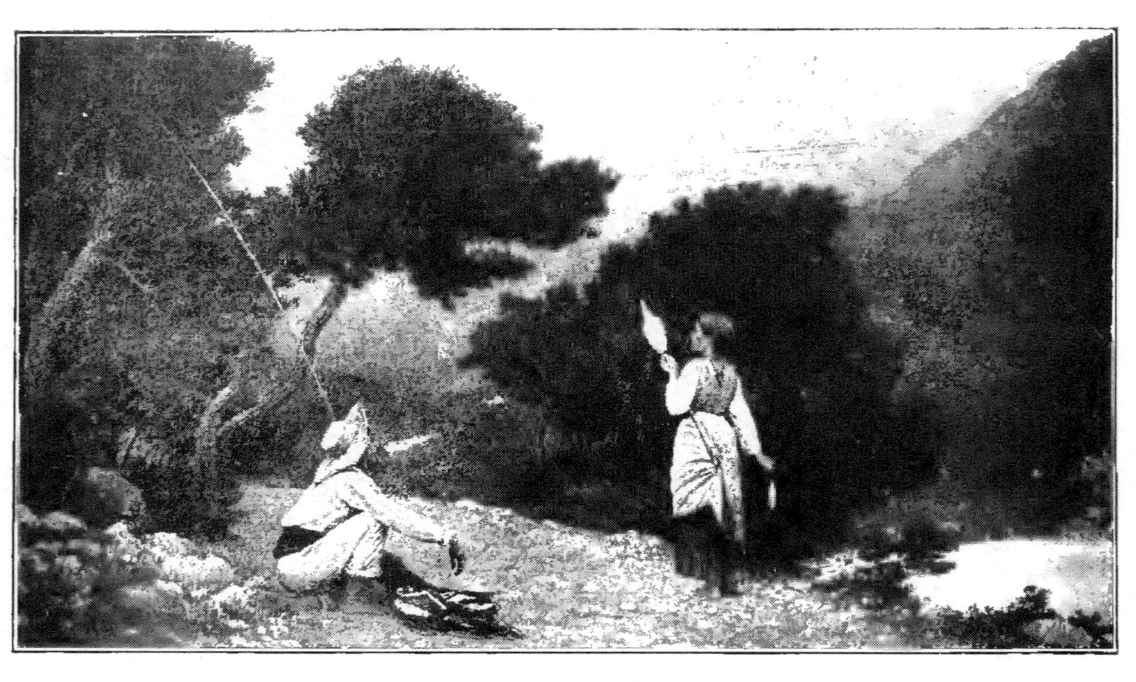

The Fisherman and Maiden
Now at Castle Howard

It may be here stated that eventually, in spite of many obstacles, the model was executed in 1885–6.

During this same visit he often met Giovanni Costa, as well as English artists who were in Rome at the time, among them Arthur Murch, Alfred Gilbert, and M. Ridley Corbet, all of whom were known to him before in England.

The above is the first reference to the series of Italian models which he was entirely instrumental in placing in the Museum. Visitors to South Kensington are familiar with these beautiful little works, and are able to gather an impression otherwise unattainable of the attraction of the originals.

There are eight of them, and a handbook published by the Department, Italian Wall Decoration of the Fifteenth and Sixteenth Centuries, gives a full account of the buildings from which the models have been reproduced. All the negotiations regarding them were personally carried out by Armstrong. They consist of .—

Chapel of S. Peter Martyr, Church of S. Eustorgio, Milan.

Chapel of S. Catherine, Church of S. Maurizio, Milan.

Appartamento Borgia, Vatican.

Appartamento in Machiavelli Palace, Florence.

Chapel in the Riccardi Palace, Florence.

Paradiso of Isabella d'Este, Ducal Palace, Mantua.

Sala del Cambio, Perugia.

Villa Madama, near Rome.

The following notes by Mr. W. M. Palin supply interesting details, and the account given later by Mr. H. Allen refers to his share in the work.

In 1882 Mr. Armstrong initiated the idea of sending the National Art Training Scholars abroad. The first experiment consisted of four of us, Thomas, Barker, Somerscales, and myself, being sent to Paris and Fontainebleau for a fortnight, to study the art decoration of the period of Francis I. and Henry II. The drawings we did from the boudoir of Marie Antoinette at Fontainebleau gave Mr. Armstrong the idea of reproducing, by models, to scale, celebrated rooms, chapels, etc., for the South Kensington Museum.

In 1883 I was the first student Mr. Armstrong sent out to Italy. I had to make measurements for, and superintend the making of, a model in wood by Milanese cabinet makers, and to copy in water-colours the frescoes and decorations by Bernardino Luini, of the chapel of S. Catherine in the Church of S. Maurizio in Milan, which were affixed to the model. I also began the reproduction of the Chapel of S. Peter Martyr in the Church of S. Eustorgio, Milan. I copied in water-colours three of the frescoes, but the difficulties that arose in obtaining permission from the church authorities to erect scaffolding necessitated the work being temporarily abandoned.

Mr. Armstrong subsequently employed Italian artists to make the models, for the reason that these permissions were more readily obtained by them.

With the exception of Mr. Herbert Allen and myself no other students carried out any reproductions.

I shall never forget the kindness and solicitude Mr. Armstrong showed with regard to my comfort. He met me in Milan, saw to my lodgings, and provided me with an introduction to an artists' club, at which I attended, without fees, a life-class two evenings a week for the whole winter. He also planned out studies for my spare time, and instructed me as to the particular art and decoration of which I should make notes and sketches.

As this was the first experiment of sending a student on his own responsibility, naturally Mr. Armstrong was keenly anxious about the result, and I am pleased to say that both he and Colonel Donnelly were satisfied. I believe several copies of the model were afterwards made by National Art Training Scholars for the provincial museums.

In 1884–5 Mr. Armstrong sent me to Rome to copy the tapestries after the designs of Raphael, which are now in the Victoria and Albert Museum : *Stoning of Stephen, Conversion of S. Paul,* and *S. Peter in Prison.* Mr. Armstrong came to Rome during the progress of my work, and again was most kind and thoughtful about my health and studies.

I should like to add that Mr. Armstrong always kept in touch with his old pupils and took the greatest interest in their welfare, and was proud of any successes they achieved.

The acquaintance with Sir George Errington begun in Rome was continued in England, and Armstrong met him often during 1884. He went with the Hon. Walter James, a painter of delicate taste, an accomplished pupil and follower of Costa's, to stay with Sir George at Lacklands, near Chippenham.

It was thought that the climate of Florida would benefit Caldecott's failing health, and he and his wife left England in October, 1885. It proved to be the breaking of this devoted and close intimacy, for news came of his dangerous illness, which made Armstrong anxious to start off for Florida at once. This report was swiftly followed by a telegram which announced his death on February 13th, 1886. An extract from a letter written at this time to Armstrong by Randolph's step-brother, the Rev. Alfred Caldecott, D.D., speaks eloquently of the relation between them :—

The friendship of you two stands out in my mind as one of the significant and real facts of human life, an expressed example of the beauty of " that most excellent gift of charity," the very bond of peace and of all virtues, humane and divine. You hardly know yourself, you cannot know, how really you were elder brother to him by a tie that makes me doubt the vaunted closeness of the bond of blood. . . . It stands manifest before all who were intimate how you " found " him, professionally speaking ; but the subtler sympathies of the inner man between you were of the nature of that profounder communion of spirit of which the pattern lies, as Plato said, " in heaven."

Armstrong arranged and sorted the work which Caldecott had left, in which their mutual friend Arthur Lemon assisted, and a sale was held at Christie's in the following June. The memorial which was erected to him in the crypt of St. Paul's is the work of Alfred Gilbert, R.A.

Armstrong naturally took a keen interest in it, and was secretary to the Memorial Committee.

In 1884 he visited the schools for the teaching of art as applied to industry at Milan, Bologna, Padua, Naples, and Florence, and his official report shows how conscientiously and thoroughly he applied himself to the discovery of what was best in the various methods of art education there practised. He concludes his report with these words: "My visits to the schools were of necessity short and somewhat hurried, but I took notes in every instance of any deviations from methods of teaching already known to me."

On another occasion when in Rome he writes: "I inspected and made notes of a number of interesting and valuable works of art now in the hands of collectors which are likely to come into the market, and which it may be desirable to acquire for the Department." Wherever he went, at home or abroad, under the heading of the locality he visited he made notes of all that might be of use either to the Museum or to the art schools, and it has been said by one of the Museum officials that these note-books have been most invaluable for reference. From Rome he writes: "I am pressing to have fresh casts made from the antique statues in the Vatican, for those which are being sold in the trade are getting blunted, and I shall not cease to press for the permission which I think so very important. I have very decided views about the supply of casts of all those works of art which can be cast without danger to the originals....Very bad casts, like many of those that have been circulated in England, are of little or no value."

The experiment of sending four students abroad, to which Mr. Palin alludes in his notes, was so encouraging that in this year the Travelling Scholarships were permanently instituted and awarded annually. Armstrong realised the difficulties that might arise to mar the profit and the enjoyment of these scholarships, for most of the students had never been abroad before, had small experience of any travel, and spoke no language but English. He therefore took the greatest pains to equip them with practical information regarding hotels, pensions, food, and locomotion, compiled from the experiences of the earlier students.

It will be readily understood that Armstrong was thoroughly in sympathy with the revival in craftsmanship led by William Morris. In an Official Report issued in 1885, on the instruction in Schools of Art, he emphasises very strongly

> the wholesome tendency of directing the student to studies which lead to contact with those trades which depend more or less on decorative art.... Without this in view the study of design will not be as helpful as those who have not well considered the matter might be led to believe; because, unfortunately, the producers of the designs are not those who can apply them, nor have they that intimate acquaintance with the practice of the workshop which should go hand in hand with artistic skill and familiarity with good examples, if truly good work is to be produced. To bring about this production of good work, we

must get hold of the artisan and make him into something of an artist, by giving him skill in drawing and modelling, and by teaching him the characteristics of styles in our schools, and especially by showing him good examples in our museums. The tradition of the workshop has been broken off, there is a constant demand for novelty....and the art workman is bewildered by the number of styles put before him; thus the necessities of life drive him to seek novelty and to sacrifice mastery.

The hurry of the times in which we live tells on our attempts to foster good art workmanship. ....The haste for immediate fruition is seen in the production of works in precious metal, such as those needed for a casket or vase intended for a royal present, which is turned out in as many weeks as it would have taken months in the hands of Benvenuto Cellini....The alternative course to making the artisan something of an artist would be inducing artists to gain familiarity, with some amount of skill, in some of the smaller arts, the processes of which were well known to many of the most famous painters and sculptors of former times....This may be difficult, but it is surely not impossible, if the idea that such work is in some way degrading or unworthy can be got over, and if the executants can get some credit for their work, and not be suppressed behind the name of the firm which acts as agent for them.

It was for the realisation of such ideas that the Arts and Crafts Society was formed, with Walter Crane as President, the first exhibition being held at the New Gallery in 1888, three years after Armstrong's official statement.

The students in whose work he took a

very great interest were the Masters in Training and the National Scholars, a group of students (workers and designers from various parts of the country) whose merit had gained them a period of scholarship at South Kensington, and who for the most part returned at the close of their scholarship to their several localities with added experience and knowledge, to the great advantage of such local industries as pottery, textile, and metal work.

These students, who were in direct contact—as workers—with industrial art production, led Armstrong to give much individual attention and supervision to their studies, for he fully appreciated the value of their work to the nation. The personal interest being so merged in the official, his influence naturally made itself potent in the Schools. All earnest workers enlisted his sympathy, which continued long after the studentship period had expired, and which showed itself whenever possible in the form of practical help and guidance. The keynote of his official attitude, or rather the idea which predominated in the shaping of his official attitude, was a profoundly conscientious regard for the fact that he was a servant of the nation, and this attitude, identifying itself with a just recognition of what was the declared object for which the Government Art Department was instituted, evidenced itself in a greater leaning to the encouragement of the practical and useful rather than of the literary, archæological, or purely theoretical. He saw in modelling clay a facile and convenient medium for the

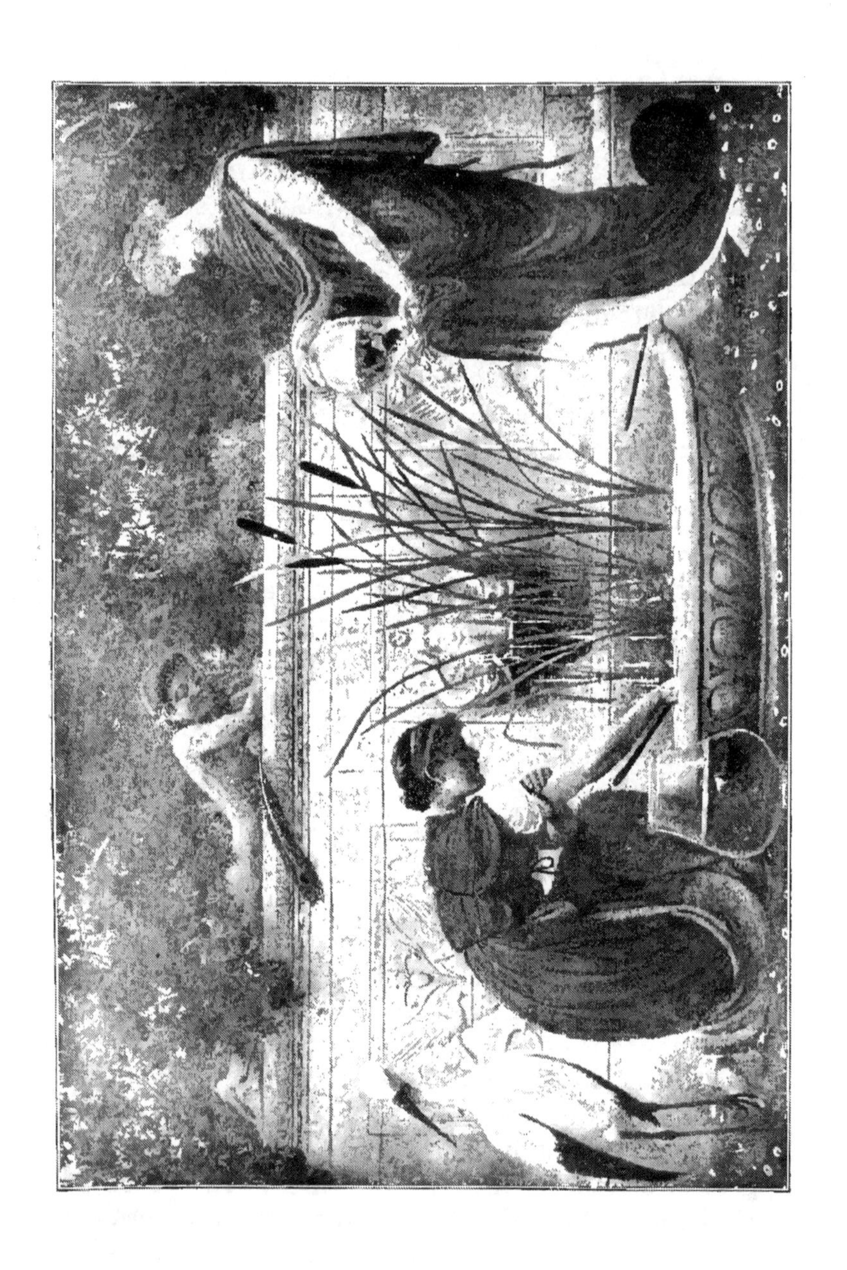

development of deftness of hand, and in the making of modelled studies of suitably selected subjects an excellent training for the eye. All this, he held, would leave its mark, whatever occupation or craft the student might afterwards be engaged in.

When he first joined the department there was little instruction in modelling, except at the National Art Training School, where Poynter had been fortunate enough to secure the services of the famous French sculptor Dalou. At the few other schools where it was taught it had quite direct application to the local industries, namely, the potteries and the great metal-work centres. The only examinations in the subject were those held at South Kensington, but under Armstrong's directorship this was changed. Arrangements were made by which any school that put forward a sufficient number of students was allowed local examinations. Under the stimulus of grants on successes the subject was taken up more and more all over the country, until, thanks to a wise application of the now discarded system of "payment on results," practically every school of any size included modelling as one of its subjects of study.

Not only so, but the specific grant offered in a special elementary modelling examination induced and enabled higher grade board schools in London and in many other places to take up the subject, with excellent results. Armstrong interested himself unceasingly in the work of the modelling school at headquarters, then under the splendid direction of Professor Lantéri, who had succeeded Dalou. The students who specialised in modelling found posts as teachers in branch and provincial schools. The enormous influence which the modelling department of the National Art Training School has had in the development of sculpture in its higher and all its subsidiary branches is one of the most striking facts relating to art education in recent times, and it had throughout the period of his directorship Armstrong's personal and official support and help.

In 1886 Armstrong was instrumental in starting the summer courses for teachers, also at the National Art Training School. These courses had proved very successful in the Science School, and Armstrong was most anxious that the provincial art masters should have the same advantages. In his official report of 1887 he says: "They were successful beyond hopes or expectations, the masters and students attending them being of necessity called together in haste....I was in the schools on most days while the courses lasted, and was much pleased with the earnestness with which the work was being done."

The course was of three weeks' duration, and given during the vacation, so that the various art masters and mistresses could attend for advanced instruction. The modelling class was under the direction of Professor Lantéri, who not only taught, but gave demonstrations before the students. Armstrong was the first to urge these being given, as he keenly appreciated their value. Lantéri has continued them ever since this date. He quotes remarks made to him by Armstrong: "It is a greater service to the country for a teacher to show a student how to make something than to talk about it"; and "Education by the eye sinks deeper than education by the ears." Demonstrations were also given in fresco-painting, casting, etc., at these summer courses. The lecturers were chosen from the leading artists, craftsmen, and designers of the day, Armstrong using his personal influence in procuring their services. He noted the needs of the students, and always endeavoured to supply them in arranging for the next courses.

In the summer of this year also a class was organised which bore far-reaching results. Armstrong's own words from a paper read to the Society of Arts in 1887 may be quoted:—

Enamel applied to metal in a coarse way for domestic utensils is common in England, and cheap, and I do not see why the finer side of the art should not be developed, especially in the jewellers' and goldsmiths' work, where its use, in a translucent form, gives effects of the greatest beauty....By the courtesy of Professor Roberts-Austen we were enabled to have the use of the metallurgical laboratory in the Science Schools at South Kensington in 1886 for a class consisting of twelve of our best students, under the instruction of M. Dalpeyrat. He was employed to make copies of some of the museum enamels, which he did most skilfully, and these copies were used for circulation among provincial museums and schools.

Each student in the class drew and painted a piece of ornament, first in opaque white on a dark ground, and afterwards heightened the effect of it with the translucent glaze over gold or silver, firing it himself in every stage. The result was very satisfactory.

At this time, it must be remembered, there was no grant for technical education. One of the twelve students was Mr. Alexander Fisher, whose distinguished work in this beautiful craft is now so prized. He contributes a brief account of his relations with Armstrong, which were, he says, of the

most cordial, not only in this respect, but throughout the term of my National Scholarship, and afterwards for many years. He was invariably kind, sympathetic, helpful, and, above all, practical. M. Dalpeyrat was a very good teacher, and knew his work thoroughly, following the Limoges enamel method, from the preparation of the plate of copper to the firing of it. Unfortunately, I was unable to attend all the class meetings, but I had enamelled on pottery before coming to London. Strange as it may appear, I am the only one of the twelve who took it up and continued to work at it. After I left the schools I was employed by the Department in copying and in tempera painting, and later I worked for about three years at enamelling at Starkie Gardner's, developing my knowledge of all the processes. I then worked with Miss Blount and Captain Ward for a short time before starting for myself, which I found a most anxious and laborious time. Mr. Armstrong then obtained for me the Tipping golden wedding presentation, which took the form of a gold and enamel casket, completed in June, 1894, and exhibited at the Academy the next year, where it was the first specimen of Limoges enamel shown for nearly a century. Through it I received many important commissions, and I can truly say I look back on Mr. Armstrong as having first given me the incentive to prosecute and develop the art. I also owed to his introduction my appointment as teacher of enamelling and silver work at the Finsbury Technical College, where I have taught most of the successful art enamellers and silver workers, including the Nelson Dawsons.

Miss Constance Blount, who at that time was very keenly interested in the Home Arts and Industries class, writes :—

Mr. Armstrong was a wonderful friend to any one who wanted to work, always ready to spend himself and to be spent in helping and advising. He had but to believe the person was conscientiously anxious to do good work and he was at his service at once. To the artisan and manufacturer he was invaluable, and many of our great firms have spoken of Mr. Armstrong's kindness in no measured terms, and have said what a boon it was to have one with the knowledge he had as Director, who was ever ready to teach and explain the difference of right and wrong principles in art or manufacture. It was not only for the successful craftsman that he exerted himself; he would be just as kind in taking round the Museum a poor potter from a country pottery, who would stand open-mouthed before the triumphs of "Maestro Giorgio," as well as appear awestruck at Mr. Armstrong's dissertations on colour and proportion. The kind Director might be a little disappointed at the lack of response from the provincial, yet he would content himself with the sight of the man's long, sensitive fingers, and afterwards, when he saw good work done, would be satisfied that his words had not been wasted. He never forgot those he thus tried to help, and often months afterwards he would come across a design or a drawing—for embossed leather, for iron, for lace, for pottery—and would say to any one he knew to be interested, "Could you get at that man for me and send him that?"

Every year great care and attention were bestowed upon the National Competition. The work of all the schools and classes receiving aid from the State is sent to South Kensington for examination, an undertaking of magnitude, as hundreds of thousands of drawings and models have to be dealt with. After a process of sifting, which goes on during two or three months, the advanced works are passed on to the special examiners. Armstrong was ever anxious to acquire the best judging, as is evidenced by the choice in the eighties of William Morris and Walter Crane to pronounce on design; Sir E. J. Poynter, George Leslie, R.A., W. F. Yeames, R.A., and Henry Marks, R.A., on figure and still-life painting; Professor George Aitchison, R.A., and Mr. J. J. Stevenson on architecture, and other well-known authorities for lace designs, machine drawing, modelling, and so on.

Commendatore Walter Crane writes:—

Armstrong was anxious to get a collective

report from the examiners upon the whole of the work in the National Competition, and with this view he invited all the examiners in different subjects to meet on one occasion, our subjects being taken rather as watertight compartments than in any real relation to each other. The examiners had also acquired the habit of regarding them and themselves in a similar spirit, perhaps; anyway I do not remember that there were any definite results from the conference, but it showed the large-minded views of Armstrong in regard to the question.

He was always anxious to record the exact words used by the examiners when they came to consider their report in any particular section. Their criticisms and remarks on the work before them are expressed verbally, and now a shorthand writer is present to take them down. I rather think Armstrong was instrumental in getting this done. The reports are typewritten and afterwards sent for correction to each examiner, so that as direct an expression of opinion as possible is obtained for the benefit of the schools.

In the examinations in Design, to which Armstrong called me in the early eighties, it was the custom to mark the papers as "excellent" or "good," or "fair" or "fail," as the case might be, defining their relative position in this way; but about 1887 a change was made, and examiners were requested to indicate the degrees of merit by numerical values; I presume, with the idea of obtaining more exact results. It was felt rather difficult to indicate the various degrees of merit in artistic capacity by means of cyphers at first, and I find a letter of Armstrong's on this subject, probably in answer to one of mine, which shows his kindly way of meeting such objections.

In the early eighties, too, I remember that Armstrong was one of the first to recognise for students of design the value of attention to the artistic handicrafts, and he got me to give a series of lectures, or rather demonstrations (in accordance with his view that clinical lectures were the only kind of value to art-students), in various crafts such as sgraffito, tempera-painting, modelling in gesso, and stencil-designing and cutting, and these were given in the Lecture Theatre at that time.

In February, 1887, Armstrong delivered the address on "The condition of Applied Art in England, and the education of the Art Workman," of which mention has already been made, before the Society of Arts, John Street, Adelphi, for which he received the silver medal.

He led his hearers through what he called "a wilderness of details about the work of the Department," and spoke of the development of art education in the country, aided by the establishment of museums, regularly fed from the rich and priceless stores of the parent collection. He emphasised the good work accomplished by the National Competition, where drawing from the human figure was ousting the highly stippled over-elaborated studies from the antique, and dwelt on the far-reaching effects of the excellent teaching in modelling instituted in the Training and other schools. His reference to enamel work has been noticed, and he mentioned as a new departure in metal work "the most interesting and beautiful Fawcett Memorial in Westminster Abbey, by one of the very best artists seen in England in our time" (Alfred Gilbert, R.A.). As regards mosaic, he saw no reason why the art should not be extensively cultivated, and it demanded attention, but he felt that there was little to be learnt about the materials and processes for making and decorating pottery. What was needed was the application of what was known "with greater judgment and discretion." He spoke of the then recently discovered frieze of enamelled pottery or majolica which adorned the Palace of Darius the Mede at Susa—the Shusan of the Book of Esther—now to be seen in the Louvre, and he hoped the decorative beauty of its form and colour would suggest possibilities of ornament on the exterior of our buildings. "Its surface is easily kept clean, but it need not be so smooth or so highly glazed as to cast unpleasant reflections." After reviewing the arts of weaving, cabinet-making, brass and iron work, and stained-glass, he briefly considered the condition of the art workman; where he again emphasises the point touched on in his Official Report regarding the artist and the artisan.

His training must begin very early in life, and if in the near future we can count on a boy coming out of a Board School with trained eyes and hands to draw with and perhaps to model, we shall be in the way of letting him profit rapidly by what he sees in Museums. Make him an artist, teach him to feel a pride in his work, and let him know that it is appreciated. Do not let him be suppressed by the dealer who sells his productions, but let his name be attached to any piece of work in which there is originality of grace or skill, or new combinations of pleasurable invention. The alternative to making the artisan into an artist is to induce the artist, as we call him, to take a turn in the workshop, and learn the craft of the artisan....In this way they acquire, if not mastery at any rate that knowledge of processes which is necessary for directing the work of others....No impetus has been given to decorative art in our time to compare with that which had its origin nearly thirty years ago in dingy Red Lion Square, where a few young men, unknown to the public but warmed by real enthusiasm, and, as the result has shown led by the light of genius, set to work quietly and without advertisement to apply Art to Industry, with the results, known to you all, associated with the name of William Morris.

Though he was often away inspecting in the country, he always found time to keep in touch with his old friends the du Mauriers, T. R. Lamont (who was often at Sheffield Gardens), Henry Wallis, Mr. and Mrs. De Morgan, Mr. and Mrs. Blackburn, and others who have been mentioned earlier. These names figure often in his diaries, in addition to the semi-official visitors and acquaintances with whom his work associated him. His geniality and excellence as a raconteur added to his true kindliness and readiness of helpful service, made him ever a most welcome guest.

In 1888 he delivered an address at the Guildhall at Cambridge, where he stayed with

Dr. Perowne at Corpus. Some of the same ground was covered as in the Society of Arts paper, and he told how " the state began to give aid to art education and the manner in which its grants to that end are now-made." There had been public criticisms implying that art teaching tended to place the workman above his trade, a point that Armstrong constantly refuted, and in this address he points out the aim of the early Select Committees who framed the scheme. In 1835 Mr. William Ewart, member for Liverpool, moved that " an inquiry be made into the best manner for extending a knowledge of the arts and principles of design among the people, especially the manufacturing population." Again in 1852, in a minute for the formation of the " Department of Practical Art," its principal objects were declared to be " instruction in drawing and modelling, and in the knowledge and practice of ornamental art, with practical application of such knowledge to the improvement of manufactures." In which schemes Armstrong said the artists proper were severely left out. He traced the history of the collection at South Kensington. Five thousand pounds was spent in purchases from the 1851 Exhibition of " objects notable ent rely for the excellence of their art or workmanship," and the educational value of a museum of decorative art applied to industry being somewhat tardily recognised, an annual vote was decided upon, which has been continued ever since. Sir Henry Cole was the central figure of the early days of the collection, and his labours were supported by able assistants, among whom Mr. J. Hungerford Pollen was em nent. Armstrong also told how the central museum serves as a store-house for the whole country, there being, as long ago as 1888 when he was speaking, thirty-three local museums, besides the more important in Edinburgh and Dublin, drawing supplies from it. "This system of circulation has not," he says, "as far as I know been practised in any other country in late years; in fact, it seems to have been in abeyance since specimens of good art-workmanship were distributed by the central authorities of ancient Egypt in Pharaonic times. Those we know of were small slabs or panels of carving in relief, and there are many in the Boulac Museum, and thanks to Mr. Henry Wallis we have now two original pieces and casts of others which are at Boulac." Later in the address he emphasises the former point noted above. "The money granted for more than fifty years in the shape of grants in aid was intended, as I have already told you, for the improvement of the art workman and designers, not to make them into artists, so called, or painters of pictures, but better workmen and better designers, so that those industries depending for commercial success on the arts of designing—those already existing and those which might be created—could hold their own against foreign competition, and thus advance the general prosperity of the country."

In April of this year, while staying near Blandford, Dorset, with his wife's relations, many

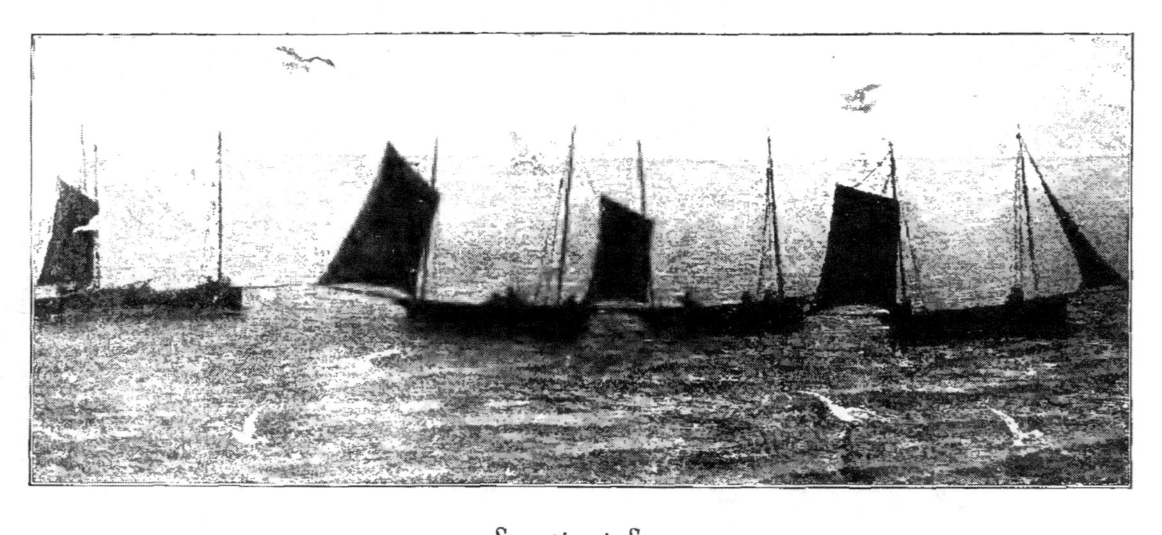

Sunset at Sea

Now at The Abbot's House

of whose ancestors were connected with that town and neighbourhood, there is an entry in his diary for the 17th which says: "Went to Blandford, where a Mr. Wyatt showed us the house in Salisbury Street where Alfred Stevens was born. Wyatt was a school-fellow of Stevens's, and is related by marriage to one Pegler of Southampton, who collected and published in a pamphlet the notices of Stevens which appeared when he died." In 1892 he was again at Charlton, and mentions going to Blandford and meeting Mr. Wyatt to look at Stevens's birth-place. He found the townspeople very apathetic about making any recognition of the great artist who had spent his boyhood amongst them, but at last through his efforts a tablet was put on the house in Salisbury Street, and a portrait in relief by Alphonse Legros has been placed in the Town Hall. Since then there has been a great awakening of interest, and the corporation of Blandford, and in particular Alderman Curtis, is properly proud of the genius who was born in their town.

After the holiday classes were once instituted, nothing was allowed to interfere with their personal supervision, so Armstrong's own vacation was always curtailed by those three weeks. In 1888 Mr. J. Hungerford Pollen was lecturing on historic ornament.

During the autumn the first Arts and Crafts exhibition was held at the New Gallery. The object of the Society, as has already been seen, met with the most cordial upholding from Armstrong, and his understanding of the aims of William

Morris and his fellow-workers was all the fuller that he also appreciated the difficulties against which they had had to contend. His admiration of Morris was unstinted, and he spoke of him as " a man who has done more than any other in our times to raise and ennoble the position of the decorative artist." The later generation who reaps the benefit of a pioneer's work fails somewhat naturally to understand the extent of its indebtedness, or to realise to what depths our decoration would have sunk without an æsthetic revival.

Early in 1889 Armstrong gave an address in Glasgow. He recapitulated the history of the instruction in Art since the State undertook the duty in 1835, and brought his remarks to bear on the present needs of the city in which he was speaking.

If you can get the artisans to your school the general well-being of your town will be promoted, for every mechanic, and especially those connected with the building trade, can be taught there something which will make his labour more valuable. For these, generally, I attach most importance to mechanical drawing with instruments—geometry, drawing to scale, and the elements of architecture. Such work is, apart from and beyond its immediate commercial value to the workman, an intellectual exercise of the highest value, inducing accurate habits of thought as well as dexterity of hand. Freehand drawing and modelling from ornament will give the clever joiner and stonemason, having perseverance and taste, a chance of becoming a carver in wood and stone, and the ordinary house-painter by such practice will be able to decorate your house with such painted ornament as is common in Italy, with profit to himself and pleasure to you.

He advocated the institution of a good Museum of industrial art, where examples of fine textiles for one thing would influence one of the chief manufactures, "but it would not be well to confine yourselves to these, for all the decorative arts, major and minor, fine and industrial, are inseparably linked together, and the influence of decorative works of what is called fine art are, in a community like yours, of inestimable value in keeping up the general standard of taste."

Official visits to Paris, where he viewed the Spitzer collection, and to Italy occupied some months of the year. While in Perugia he was making arrangements for the model of the Sala del Cambio. Mr. W. Herbert Allen, a former student, and now Head Master of the School of Art at Farnham, contributes an account of his connection and correspondence with Armstrong.

The greater number of my letters refer to business matters connected with my work for the Museum, and more especially to the series of models. Mr. Armstrong watched the progress of these works with intense interest, and was keenly alive to the artistic bearing of everything, down to the most minute parts. Many letters were written to me whilst at work in Paris and in various Italian cities, and they all testify in a marked manner to that rare and kind solicitude which he never failed to exhibit towards those of us who were working for the Museum and teaching under the Department. The earlier letters were written to me when in Italy in 1889 with Mr. A. C. Jahn (now the Head Master of the Sheffield School of Art). We had both won travelling scholarships in the previous year, and the letters contain much valuable counsel as to how we should best employ our time and what we should study. I came to Farnham in the autumn of 1889, and subsequently did some decorative work, coloured lacquer upon gold and silver foils, for Mr. Armstrong. In 1892 I was sent to Florence to execute the little model of the Machiavelli Palace. It consisted of the rendering of a portion of a room dated about 1350 with its original decorations, the room and old palace to which it belonged now incorporated in Signor Bardini's gallery. In 1895 I was engaged in painting my model of the Riccardi Chapel in Florence when I received instructions to go to Mantua to meet M. Yriarte, to inspect and make a report upon the series of apartments known as the Paradiso of Isabella d'Este. Mr. Armstrong wrote that he had long thought it desirable to have a model of the room for which pictures were painted by Mantegna, Perugino, and others. Isabella's letters ordering these paintings are still extant, though some of the pictures themselves are now in the Louvre. It was wished, to make it complete, to have these pictures copied and attached to the model in their original positions, in order faithfully to reproduce the effect of the whole as at first designed. He assured me that I should find M. Yriarte, who was a personal friend, very pleasant and instructive to work with, as his knowledge of Italian art was profound. M. Yriarte explained to me that he had found Mantua so rich a subject that he had expanded his work into two volumes, one on the city, and the second on Mantegna. I made a rather interesting little discovery in the Paradiso. A gleam of bright sunlight upon the floor of the room had sent so brilliant a ray through a hole in one of the pictures (the inferior ones now occupying the positions of those represented in my model) that it revealed a fine piece of Mantegnesque decoration on the wall at the back. M. Yriarte had the pictures temporarily removed, but the decoration uncovered was evidently of the nature of an experiment, subsequently abandoned. I was at work in Paris in 1896 on the copies of the Paradiso pictures, and Mr. Armstrong interested himself about the media in which ease and quality of work were best attained. The whole of his letters over many years were all inspired by the most kindly feeling, and an intense personal concern in matters connected with his art. Nothing that had merit escaped his notice.

Mention should be made of Mr. Armstrong's practical interest in the students' sketching club at the Royal College of Art, to which he was accustomed to give two prizes a year, both during his directorate and in his retirement. One was for a decorative panel of a given subject, such as commerce, labour, autumn, etc., and the second for the best set of studies of growing plants. He used to urge us to make rapid sketches of people working in the fields, quarrying, making pottery, and so on.

Mr. Armstrong used to dwell very strongly in regard to pictorial art on the necessity of giving the utmost consideration to the decorative value of the composition as a whole. He would speak of the pains with which Leighton would arrange his subject; in the first place in little drawings, wherein he would arrive at a precise decision as to the proportion and relation of the figure or figures to the area of the enclosing rectangle. Mr. Armstrong would go on to remind us of the value and grandeur of fine silhouettes, and also say that in his opinion a picture should so far as colour was concerned, have a definite complexion, so that one picture might be a blue picture, another a green. He felt, I think, that in pictorial work decorative considerations should be paramount. I recall one evening, when Fisher and I were dining with him, and I had mentioned an exceedingly beautiful and apt verse by which one of our students had entitled a decorative frieze illustrating "Harvest," he replied with a smile, "How much better it would be if you fellows did not know how to read."

Stress, I think, should be laid on the fact that although, as was fully evinced by all his work, Mr. Armstrong was eminently classic in his predilections, his tendency, perhaps owing to his being a painter, inclined him to admire and advocate early Italian art of the Renaissance rather than actual classic work. It was, I am sure, owing chiefly to him that examples of the art of the before-mentioned period came to be prominently set before students in England. I refer chiefly to the work of Donatello, of Rosellino, Luca della Robbia, and Desiderio da Settignano.

It was a little before this time that the *Angelus* of J. F. Millet fetched such a sensational price, and mention of this picture in a letter to Armstrong from John Bancroft is worth noting.

Did I tell you of my special interest in the *Angelus*, of which its stupendous value has again reminded me? In the spring of 1859 I left Dresden for Düsseldorf, and then by a sudden inspiration (fruitless of result, however) started in search of the unknown in the shape of a summer of Barbizon, a convert from German heresies as soon as I arrived. The *Angelus* was finished that summer, and I saw it on Millet's easel a day or two after the last touches, and coveted it, though of narrow means. I tried to buy it, but learned that it was (supposed to be) sold to a countryman of mine, no name given, for two thousand francs. And so ended my short negotiation. The next winter was that pleasant one in Düsseldorf*, and when we all scattered in the following spring, I went to Paris to stay. At the house of common friends I met a compatriot, well known to me by name, for the first time. We left the house together, and strolling down the street, he, much my senior, questioned me kindly, talked of art, then of Barbizon, of Millet, and finally of the *Angelus*. He told me (as if I enjoyed it !) how he had seen it while painting, and had said to Millet that he had never seen a picture he would sooner wish to own, and how Millet had understood this friendly sympathy as an order for the picture, and what difficulty he had met with to avoid having a picture forced on him which he meant to praise only, but not to buy. All this charmingly told, but, you see, to the wrong person, who could get no enjoyment at all out of the confidence. Years passed on, and the picture became famous. I saw my amateur from time to time, and he was conscious of a frostiness between us. With the growing fame of the picture his mind underwent a delightful transformation, until one day I heard him tell his story again. This time it ran that the hope of his life had been to leave this great picture at

* The time of the meeting with du Maurier and Armstrong.

his death to the Boston Museum ; it had been his, ordered by him of Millet when half done, the price agreed upon, and never delivered in spite of his persistent efforts and inquiries. He died a few years ago, and all his family and friends except myself are firmly persuaded that he was defrauded of the ownership. There was one short chapter in the story which he never told, but which I heard from a brother of Millet's. He made a second visit to Barbizon, and presented himself at the studio as a stranger wishing to see the artist and his work. The tale goes that Millet courteously invited him to come in, and then asked him if he were not the same Mr. A. who had visited him on a picture-buying errand a year or two before, and on his confession of identity, with majestic gesture, " Voilà la porte ! " the curtain falls.... The real reason, you see, why the *Angelus* did not come to Boston for two thousand francs and no duties (a modern invention) was my being in that remote village of Düsseldorf while all this was going on unknown to me.

The official work in 1890 included prize-giving, with an address, at Birmingham. He naturally applied himself to local needs when making these speeches, as the following extract shows:

There are two classes to whose improvement in the matter of art-education I look with great interest. With regard to one of them, I am not sanguine ; nay, I almost despair of winning them —I mean the young men of the upper or wealthier classes. If these could be got to learn drawing seriously, useful drawing, in their school-days as they learn writing, and could be induced to interest themselves in architecture and the other attendant or ancillary arts, we should soon have a leverage in a body of public opinion which would make itself felt. It is especially with reference to those young people of wealthy parents, who are destined to control the large firms engaged in industries depending on the arts of design for success, that I make this suggestion; and for these it is desirable that their course of instruction should begin early, should be conducted seriously, and on sound principles, and be carried far. From what I saw and heard lately in North Germany, where there is great activity to rival and displace English wares, I am convinced that it is not by trying to instruct the artisan only that we shall hold our own or extend our borders. We must cultivate those who by inheritance succeed to control in these firms, or who are likely to become highly paid directors or managers.

The other class is more under control—I mean the children in the Board Schools—and I think that here in Birmingham, where the way is being shown, I shall have your sympathy and approval when I express my most sanguine, earnest desire to have useful drawing properly taught in all elementary schools and with sufficient time given to its study....This seems to me by far the most important and most urgent art-question of the day, leading to and included in what is called technical education. The difficulty lies in the crowding out of drawing by the multifarious subjects which are now taught. For drawing, a minimum of an hour and a half a week is required, and it is hardly possible to have much more, for the day cannot be lengthened and the powers of endurance in the children cannot be increased. If, however, it should be generally recognised that drawing is almost of equal value with reading, writing, and arithmetic, and is second to no other subject taught as a preparation for the business of life among those who work with their hands for a living, and three hours a week at least were compulsorily devoted to its study in every school, as in Birmingham, I believe that in three or four years we should see a marvellous change in the work produced in our Schools of Art and art classes.... If the inevitable drudgery which must be gone through can be passed early in childhood, like that we have all gone through in learning to read and write, and if even the requirements of the Fourth Standard only can be met before the boy leaves the elementary school, he will go to the night class sufficiently prepared to begin work which will interest him, and will do it with a good heart....Improvement in the teaching of drawing in elementary schools is the highway to that technical education which is now so much desired. In a lecture delivered last year a friend of mine spoke with wonder and something of reprobation at Aristotle having said, "Reading and writing and the art of design are taught for their serviceableness in purposes of life and their precious utility." For my part I should be glad if Aristotle's views obtained more generally in the present day.

Meetings and consultations were held with Mr. Tate concerning his proposed gift of pictures to the nation, and an autumn visit was paid to Italy; there was besides, of course, his immediate work at South Kensington and the usual holiday course of lectures.

For some time past Armstrong and his wife

had been looking for a house in the country, and they finally decided in August upon buying The Abbots House, at Abbots Langley, in Hertfordshire. It had undoubtedly belonged in the old days to the Abbot of St. Albans, together with some monastic buildings which have long since disappeared, but foundations of which are still occasionally unearthed when alterations are made in the grounds.

As far back as the time of Edward the Confessor the great tithes of the parish had been granted to the Abbot of St. Albans as a provision for the clothing of the brothers, and this house and its predecessor were both most probably used by the Abbot or his agent when collecting his dues. The old inhabitants of the village still speak of the top floor, now divided into attics, as "the monks' storehouse." After the Reformation it became a farmhouse, and early in the eighteenth century was altered to its present state. In a round space below the cornice in front of the house Armstrong placed a relief, the profile bust of an abbot, his hand raised in the act of blessing, the features being those of Dr. Festing, then Bishop of St. Albans, brother of his colleague, Major-General Festing.

Social and official life ran its course until a baleful interruption came in January, 1892, when in one of the severe epidemics of influenza the whole family, in fact the whole household at Sheffield Gardens, was laid low. Armstrong was seriously ill, but in course of time recovered, though his health was never so secure as before this attack. The result of the illness on the little son Ambrose, now nine years old, was more grave, and his condition became so delicate that school had to be given up, and he spent much of the year with his mother at Abbots Langley. To escape the severity of the following winter Ambrose was taken to Algiers, where his father's old friend, George Howard, now Earl of Carlisle, was staying with one of his daughters when Mrs. Armstrong and the boy first went. The whole of 1893 was a time of great anxiety, which increased as the year drew to a close, and in April of 1894, when his eleventh birthday had just passed, Ambrose died in Sheffield Gardens. The pathos of the breaking of his short, happy life may only be touched upon. Until that terrible attack of influenza this fine and beautiful little boy had ailed nothing.

In the neighbourhood of the Abbots House is Breakspear's farm, where Adrian IV., Nicholas Breakspear (died 1159), the only English Pope, was born. This afforded Armstrong an opportunity of carrying out one of the gracious little acts in which he delighted, and he had a water-colour sketch made of the view from the farm, which was presented by Monsignor Stonor to Leo XIII., who hung it in his private apartments. Monsignor Stanley, brother to Lady Carlisle, was to have made the presentation, but he had been recalled to England by the illness of his mother, Lady Stanley of Alderley.

Early in 1895 Mr. Arthur Acland, who had been appointed Vice-President of the Council of Committee on Education, wished to make numerous alterations in the syllabus issued by the Science and Art Department. A lengthy conference of inspectors was held to consider his suggestions, and there was much difference of opinion over the alternative syllabus. Altogether it was a most trying and anxious time, the strain of which seriously affected Armstrong's health. But he could never be induced to put aside work, and when unable to go to his office he transacted business and interviewed people at his own house.

In July he attended Huxley's funeral, for whom he had always entertained the warmest feeling of regard.

In 1896 there were grievous breaches made by the death of many friends of long standing, and so much sadness retarded his own return to health. In January Lord Leighton died, in the same month that his peerage was confirmed, and Armstrong attended his funeral at St. Paul's. He felt deeply this ending of a long and most sympathetic friendship. In June his colleague, Dr. Middleton, Director of the Museum, died under sad circumstances, and Mr. (afterwards Sir) Caspar Purdon Clarke was appointed in his place. In August Mr. R. Courtenay Bell died suddenly, the host of so many pleasant gatherings. Sir John Millais died also in August, after very pathetic sufferings, leaving the office of President of the Royal Academy vacant for the second time in eight months. The appointment of Sir E. J. Poynter as Millais's successor was a great pleasure to Armstrong, and the several old friends were amused to think that the initials "P.R.A.," appended in fun to a drawing of Poynter by du Maurier in 1855, were prophetic.

In their intermittent visits to England Armstrong always saw his old friend John Bancroft and his wife and family. They corresponded regularly, and in a letter of February of this year, after reference to some Chinese vases which had been on loan at the Museum—his collection of oriental china and prints was most valuable and remarkable—he goes on to say referring to the success of *Trilby*:—

You ought certainly to write *your* recollections of Paris and du Maurier. To meet your objections to the labour of writing, I think I have a happy suggestion to make: that you and Lamont should come together and tell tales to one another and warm one another up, and have a shorthand writer in the corner of the room. I cannot but think that you would without much effort and quite spontaneously produce something very original in form and interesting.

But it was in October that the loss which so closely affected him fell, for George du Maurier, the loved and valued friend of over forty years, died in London on the 8th. There had never been any break in the intimacy begun in Paris between these two and Lamont, and as the years passed events only cemented the friendships by many sympathetic bonds.

William Morris died but a few days previously, and Armstrong went to the funeral at Kelmscott.

He was much struck, as were all present, by the beautiful simplicity of the ceremony. A yellow farm waggon, fine in form, wreathed and lined with boughs and moss, carried the oak coffin from Lechlade station to the churchyard, drawn by a strong, sleek horse, and led by one of the carters.

His old friend Henry Blackburn died at Bordighera in March, 1897, with whom and his circle lay so many associations.

Some drawings sent from the West Ham School of Art attracted his attention as being the work of a boy of nine. Their excellence was so marked that he had special inquiries made about them, which resulted in his sending for the boy. As a consequence he arranged that Newbury Trent should come as often as possible on Saturday afternoons to draw at the Museum from objects chosen by Armstrong himself. This is an instance of the extreme care and solicitude that he showed when a promising student came under his notice. The interest in this case became a personal one on both his and Mrs. Armstrong's part, for the boy was invited every year to spend large parts of his holidays at The Abbots House, and the utmost help was given him in fostering his natural gifts. Their kindly interest was justified by his success, for he took prizes every year he was at the Training School, and at nineteen he was in the second place for drawing from the life in the whole kingdom, and also a Royal Exhibitioner.

Towards the end of the year he received a letter from Lord Salisbury saying that the

Companionship of the Order of the Bath was to be conferred on him in recognition of his many services, and his name appeared among the New Year honours of 1898. Congratulations poured in, and from those friends who had reason to know how trying and even harassing his official life had been rendered for the last few years a particular cordiality was noticeable. They felt that the honour was a deservedly opportune recognition of his earnest work for the Department.

His close and intimate friend T. R. Lamont died in April, after several weeks' illness, during which time he had been full of anxiety and hoping for his recovery. He performed the last service for this friend, as he had done for du Maurier, by attending the cremation at Woking, and in both cases showed his devotion by personal and sympathetic help to those who were mourning.

In July he went to Windsor Castle for the investiture of his Companionship, and with the other recipients of various honours was entertained at luncheon in St. George's Hall. On 1st August he opened the last of the holiday classes instituted by him, and on the 19th closed and said a few words of farewell to the students. On October 9th comes the entry in his diary: "End of my official service in Science and Art Department." He received the following letter from Sir John Gorst, who had succeeded Mr. Acland as Vice-President :—

I am very sorry to hear from Donnelly that the time has actually arrived when our official connection ceases. I am glad for your sake that

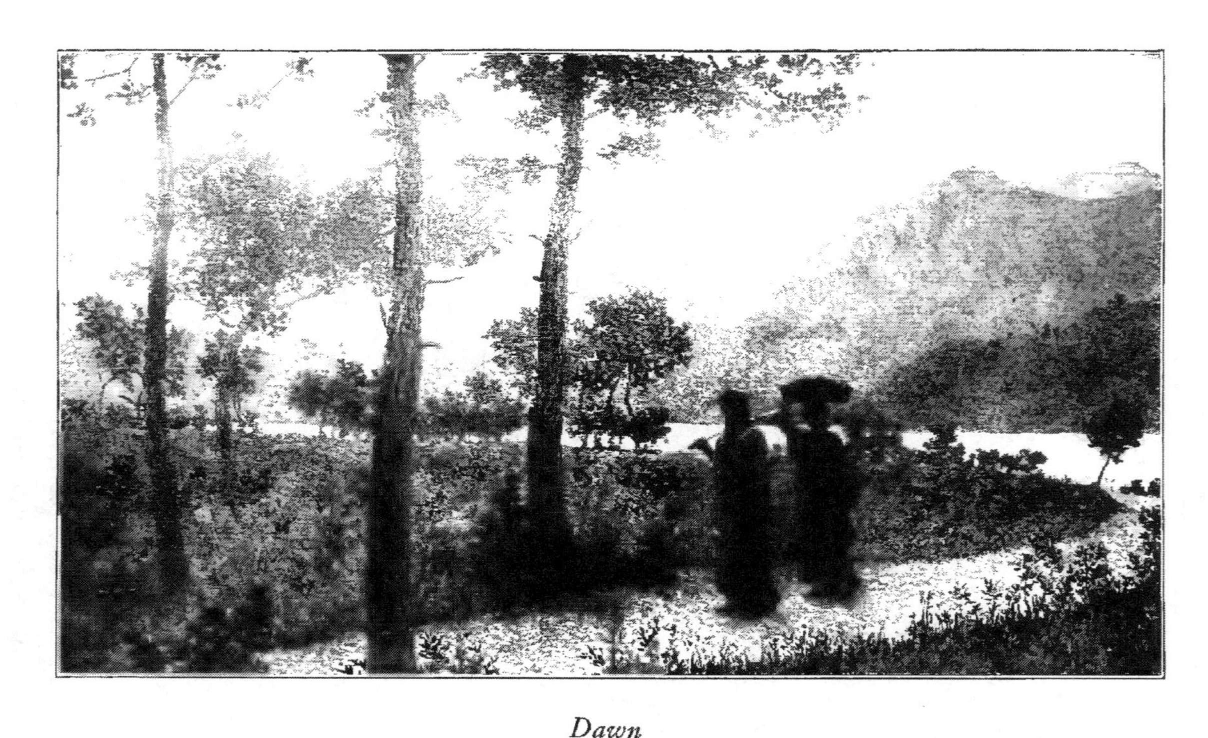

Dawn

From a Study of the Mountains behind Mentone, 1908
Now at The Abbot's House

you will have some well-earned leisure at the close of your long and valuable public services, but partıng is always melancholy. I feel personally very grateful to you for the courtesy and consideration you have always shown me during our official connection, and I hope you will long live to enjoy your rest.

Strictly speaking, by age limit his term had come to an end twelve months previously, but he was asked by Sir John Gorst if he would continue in his office for another year, as owing to the commission of inquiry into the Museum affairs matters were in a state of transition. He still attended at his office for a few weeks, as he was anxious to leave papers and correspondence in good order

After his retirement he continued to work occasionally for the Department, both in inspections and in the giving of expert opinion on objects offered to the Museum

He received many tributes of regret upon his resignation, and tributes also of a more substantial nature. A bookcase, made of the size and design to suit his wishes, and bearing the inlaid inscription, "From his colleagues in the Department of Science and Art," was presented to him, containing the *Encyclopædia Britannica*, and also Littré's *Dictionnaire de la Langue Française;* while the Art Masters and Students in Training gave a beautiful gilded and enamelled lamp.

On his retirement residence in town was given up, much to Mrs. Armstrong's satisfaction, for when life in London had come to such a sad end at Sheffield Gardens in 1894 she had never felt able to take it up again, and found country occupations more congenial to her. She was glad to be able to rearrange the pleasant rooms of The Abbots House with the rest of the furniture from town, and make it more comfortable for the many relatives and old friends it was so great a pleasure to them both to entertain.

Armstrong's leisure for several years past had been devoted to work on a monument to be erected to the memory of Ambrose in Abbots Langley Church. The following is his own account of it :—

The mural monument on the north wall of the parish church was designed, and for the most part executed by me. My main idea was to do two panels of scripture subjects in low relief, coloured after the manner of the work of the Italian artists of the sixteenth century. The figure subjects were modelled in plastelline and then cast in plaster, to be finished by carving with steel tools, a very laborious process. I made experiments with other materials, but at last I had the final casts made with plaster mixed with a kind of cement. These were coloured with tempera, and when the rest of the monument was finished were put up in the church.

After some years I found that the surface of the panels was perishing, and was degraded by the condensation, mixed with dust, running down the face of them ; to wash them was impossible. After I was seventy I resolved to do the two panels again. They were originally representations of what is called the Riposo, or

Rest on the Flight into Egypt, and the Massacre of the Innocents. Concerning the latter, by this time my feelings had changed, and I made up my mind to substitute for it Joseph and Mary finding Christ in the Temple. The composition of the Riposo, too, was altered in order to make the figures rather larger and more agreeable in their scale. The process of work was much the same as in the earlier panels, casts in plaster being taken from clay or plastelline models, worked on afterwards with steel tools. When these were finished I had copper electrotypes made from them, and on these I painted with oil colours, the surface of which would bear washing.

The colour of these is not nearly so agreeable as that of the tempera paint used for the earlier panels, but I believe it will last without deterioration.

The portrait head in the middle of the monument is in alabaster. The two figures on the top of the cornice were modelled from my drawing by Miss Levick (now Mrs. Gervase Bailey), and after being cast in plaster had copper deposited on them, and over this gold leaf was applied. The two figures represent the boy's two godfathers, T. R. Lamont, the water-colour artist, and the Earl of Carlisle, and are as far as possible portraits, indeed Lord Carlisle gave Miss Levick a sitting. He is represented as St. George slaying the dragon, and Lamont as St. Ambrose writing the "Te Deum," the boy's names having been Ambrose George. The carving of the frame was done by the teachers of the School of Art Wood Carving, and was offered as a contribution from them to the memorial.

The legends are in Latin, because I thought that by this means I should avoid as far as possible giving a personal character to the monument.

Although I must admit that the time and labour spent on the Abbots Langley panels is out of all proportion to the result, I think it might be possible to achieve a much more satisfactory result with different materials. Alabaster occurs to me as most suitable, and the carving of it would not have been more costly in labour than my cast and chiselled plaster, or the deposited copper on which I was obliged to fall back in my last extremity. The colouring, I think, must be done with tempera, which would require to be renewed from time to time, though I believe that some approach to the quality of tempera might be secured by very dry oil paint (zinc white being used) laid on with benzine. In the ambulatory of Amiens Cathedral there are a number (eight, I think) of compositions of figures about a foot high, some in relief and others round, which have interested me very much, and I think something of that kind is worth trying for. When Alfred Gilbert's mural monument to Mr. Fawcett in Westminster Abbey was being done, I admired the little figures very much, but I think the colouring has suffered from exposure to the atmosphere. It is not difficult to produce an agreeable and durable effect with tempera on small figures which can be protected by glass.

There is in the Victoria and Albert Museum a cast of the beautiful Robbiana Madonna (attributed to Luca), which has been coloured by my friend Mr. David McGill in a manner entirely novel. The colour (oil) was copiously diluted with spirit and applied as a spray.

When it was freshly done I thought it the most satisfactory specimen of coloured statuary

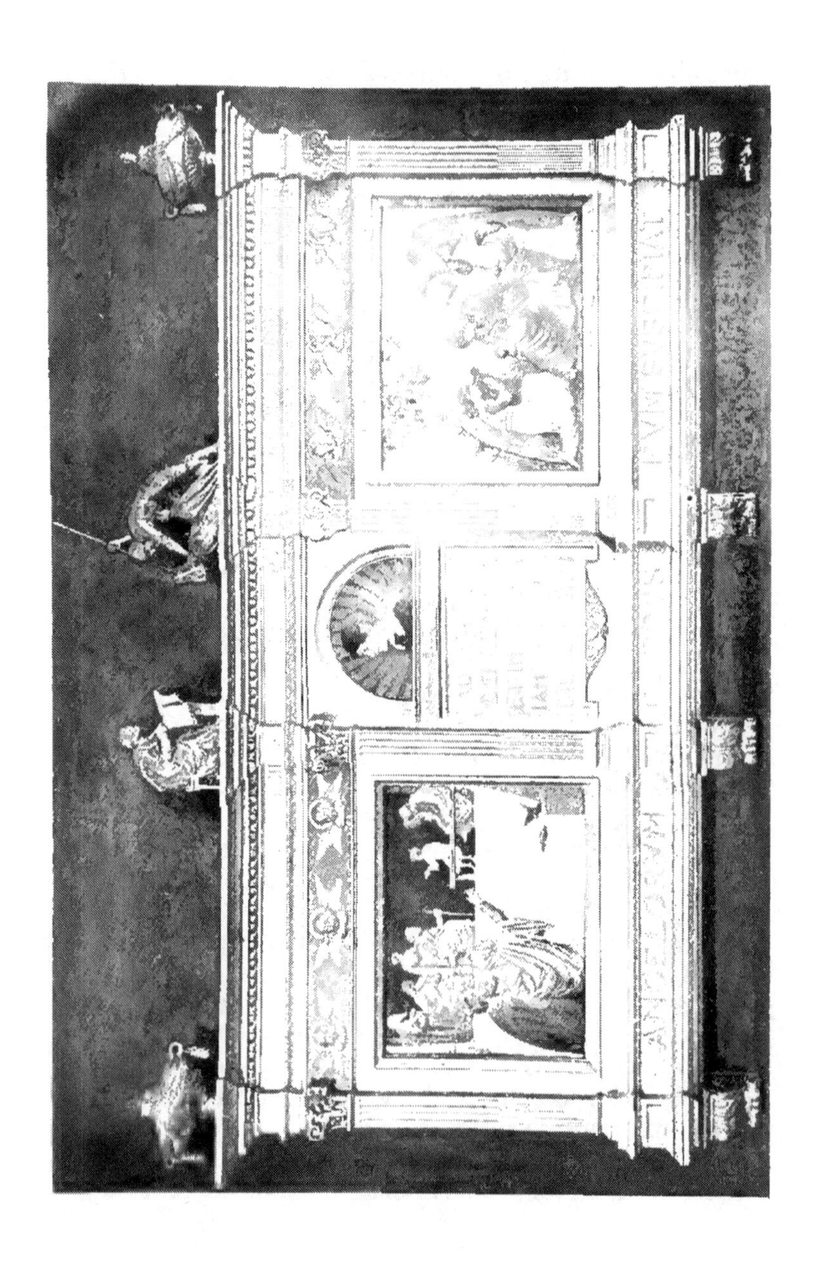

I had ever seen, but much of its charm has been lost through the effect of the lime in the plaster on the pigments used.

Mention has not yet been made of his connection with the School of Art Woodcarving. Miss Rowe, who was for so many years its manager, kindly furnishes the following account :—

Shortly after his official appointment at South Kensington Mr. Armstrong was induced by the late Sir John Donnelly, Chairman, to join the Committee of the School of Art Woodcarving. This school was started in 1878 by The Society of Arts , the Chairman, Sir John, at that time Colonel, Donnelly, took the very keenest interest in it, and never lost an opportunity of introducing on the committee any one whose advice and experience would be of benefit in its development. He remained chairman until his death in April, 1902, when, by a unanimous vote of the Committee, Mr. Armstrong was appointed to succeed him in the office, which he also retained until his death. He fully emulated the whole-hearted zeal of his predecessor, and the successful development of the school, which was the first Craft School to be started in London, is mainly due to the personal interest and supervision of its first two chairmen. Mr. Armstrong filled the position perfectly, as his kindly humour was irresistible and his judgment unerring. He was always courteous, patient, and tactful, and successfully piloted the affairs of the school through many a difficult crisis. During the twenty-nine years that he was connected with it, he was only once absent from a meeting of the committee. He constantly visited the school, and many commissions for work were obtained through his influence, and superintended by him with the keenest interest. He did a great deal to revive the use of carved and gilded frames, and had several of the water-colours under his charge at the Museum reframed and the white mounts taken away.

He was of opinion that in the Technical Schools too much insistence was laid on combining literary with art education, and in a letter dated January, 1911, he writes: "It is hoped that the L.C.C. will not press its demands for the addition of a course of literary instruction to be added to the curriculum of the school, but will be satisfied if we turn out good woodcarvers, as we have in the past. We appreciate the humanity of the Council's proposals to improve the general education of our pupils, and thus make them good citizens, but with the short time now allowed for the period of pupilage, and with our restricted means....we think we could not hope for success in adding book learning to our courses of instruction."

The Staff at the School of Art Wood Carving say they owe much to his unfailing sympathy and kindness, as well as to his excellent taste and judgment. At home or abroad, if he saw anything likely to help the student a note of it was at once made. The keen interest with which he supervised every detail of the work in the school had a marked influence on those teachers and students who had the privilege of being brought into personal contact with him.

There was another branch of artistic work in which Armstrong was much interested, and upon which he was often consulted, namely, the designing of memorials for friends, which were both simple and elaborate. He felt strongly that the usual selection of white marble was most unsuitable for this climate, which led him to employ wood, iron, and certain kinds of stone. When the memorials were to be erected under cover he made free use of beautifully coloured marbles, gilding, and enamel. The most striking examples of these are the font erected to the memory of Mrs. Charles Hunter Stewart in Edinburgh, and the mural tablet to Lady Green in York Minster. He also designed a dignified monument to William Coltart in Birkenhead cemetery in Hopton-wood stone. In all of these he availed himself of Newbury Trent's help, whose careful training was developing his rich natural gifts.

Though he had retired officially, he kept in touch with matters of keen interest to him as long as his health permitted.

The last month of 1899 and early part of 1900 Armstrong and his wife spent in Italy and the Riviera. During their stay in Naples they saw their friend Miss Blount constantly, and her congenial tastes and her hospitality made their time there memorably enjoyable. Though they had not met very frequently in later years, it was a grief to him to learn of the death of John Bancroft in Boston. They had so many tastes in common to unite them. Armstrong wrote an appreciative article, " An Artist in Woodwork," in The Art Journal of April, 1902, on his friend's craftsmanship. He worked in the Moorish manner, and " the small panels forming the ground behind his entrelacs were often elaborately inlaid, and the mouldings themselves occasionally relieved with fine lines of brass let into the wood." He goes on to explain Bancroft's method of work, and says: "He pushed his art, one would be tempted to say, to the limits of perfection."

His own health was precarious in 1902, and it was another year of losses to him, affecting him nearly. Two of his fellow workers died, Sir John Donnelly and John Hungerford Pollen, with both of whom his relations had always been most intimate and affectionate; and his friend Mathew Ridley Corbet, A.R.A., died in June, after a short illness. His brother, Frederick Armstrong, had come to London from Milan in July, very ill, and lived only till October, Armstrong devoting every possible care and attention to him. His ashes are buried in Abbots Langley churchyard, near the spot where Ambrose and his father lie.

Armstrong and his wife paid visits every year, usually in the winter, to Torquay, to visit Colonel and Mrs. Brine, and cousins of Armstrong's in other parts of the county. And in these latter years they stayed often at South Lytchett Manor, where his cousin Sir Eliott Lees lived. Armstrong enjoyed sketching in that country, the effects of light and shadow over the Poole estuary making a strong appeal to him.

Whistler died in July, 1903, and though of late years Armstrong and he had met but seldom there had been no estrangement, and he felt it was yet another break with the associations dating from the mid-fifties.

From time to time he worked in town, when he needed models, which were mostly for his renewed work on the Monument. He sometimes had the use of friends' studios. One year it was Mrs. De Morgan's, and another it was Miss Levick's (Mrs. Gervase Bailey). He and Lord Carlisle met often, either at Palace Green or at Abbots Langley. In March, 1906, he and his wife and a young friend, Miss Reid, who had been a school-fellow of Ambrose's, and to whom they were much attached, went for a fortnight's visit to Paris. He did not feel well there, and very soon after his return developed pneumonia, and was most dangerously ill. Gradually, however, he made a good recovery, and spent his convalescence at South Lytchett.

As the months went on he went less often to town for the day, as it fatigued him, but he paid occasional short visits to intimate friends in London, Mrs. du Maurier, Mrs. Westlake, and Mrs. Corbet among them.

In the summer and autumn longer visits were often paid to old friends. He and his wife stayed with Mr. and Mrs. Phipson Beale in Scotland, with Sir Edward Green at York, with Mr. and Mrs. John Kennedy (she had been Miss Ethel Reid) at Charmouth, and also at Birkenhead with his very old friend Mrs. Coltart (who was formerly Mrs. Tong); and there were many others. The revival of old associations always gave him the keenest pleasure.

In the autumn of 1908 he was very grieved at the death of his cousin Sir Eliott Lees, after only a few days' illness. His loss made a sad blank in the affectionate intercourse so long maintained with him and his family.

In the following year, while staying at Torquay, he again fell gravely ill of pneumonia, with complications, and his state was most critical; but his naturally good constitution asserted itself, and, to quote Mrs. Armstrong's words, "he gradually regained some measure of health." He needed to be careful, and had to think about "resting" a good deal.

In June of 1909 King Edward opened the new buildings at South Kensington, henceforth to be known as the Victoria and Albert Museum, and Armstrong was well enough to be present. It was a stately and imposing ceremony.

His advice or opinion was frequently sought concerning works of art of all kinds, and he took an especially keen interest in the preservation of pictures. While visiting friends, he always examined their paintings, and, whenever possible, did what might be required himself, taking great trouble in cleaning and varnishing them, for he was proud of having been taught to carry out this process thoroughly when a student at Antwerp.

He continued always to keep a diary, recording his doings quite briefly; and the entry for 6th October of this year reads: "Worked all day at my MSS. with Miss Rowe, and after she had gone I finished arranging them." He had not felt strong enough since his illness in the winter to work much in his studio, and he had occupied many of the "resting" hours prescribed by the doctor in making notes of his student days, and of the friends and events of passed years. They form the next section of this book. When they were finished the manuscript was given to his god-daughter, Mrs. Charles Hoyer Millar, the eldest daughter of George du Maurier, as they contained so much about her father, and it is by her kind permission they are now published. The writing was an interest and amusement to him which he could follow without taxing his strength.

He writes in December to an old friend abroad—Mme. Chassériaux, the Miss Bell of the far-off Algiers days of 1858 :—

From time to time I have made notes of the life I led in Paris with du Maurier, Whistler, and Poynter, and I have spent much time in trying to put these into some sort of order for publication. But I have put off doing this too long, and I feel that I have not made the narrative so interesting as I could have done twenty or even ten years ago. However, I have some unpublished drawings by du Maurier, done in 1857, of our confraternity, and these may help to make the text interesting.

But during the autumn of this year, in spite of ill-health, he designed his last piece of decorative work, and in great part executed it himself. It was a frieze of seagulls for Mrs. John Kennedy's drawing-room—a charming scheme of colour with some quaint and effective details. In a letter to Miss Lees he writes :—

Lately I have been in a more active state,

and have just finished a frieze of flying birds.... to go round Ethel's drawing-room. I have a "curate" (as Burne-Jones used to call his assistant)—a lady in the village*—who has helped me before, and she has done much of the painting under my eye, and done it very well too. It was rather a mad thing to undertake at my age, but somehow it has got itself done, and I am rather proud.

He spent many days at intervals in 1910 sorting papers and letters, the accumulation of many years and many events. He writes again to Mme. Chassériaux in December :—

I am feeling a good deal older than I did a year ago, but I have much to be thankful for, although I am living a more and more retired country life, for I do not go to London very often. ....I still potter about in my studio and make believe that I am an artist. It gives me satisfaction and does nobody any harm.

As must inevitably happen, gaps were made in long-standing friendships. Professor George Aitchison, R.A., with whom associations stretched back to the time of his first living in London, died in May, 1910, and Mrs. Armstrong's father, Colonel Brine, died in the same month, after a short illness. Early in 1911 Frederic J. Shields died, after suffering terribly for years from ill-health, though he had lived to finish his remarkable work in the Chapel of the Ascension, Bayswater. Armstrong was not himself well enough to attend the funeral, for the year began with very poor health. But he recovered sufficiently to benefit by a visit to Chichester, and in March

* Miss Teresa Sadler.

was in Devonshire. He was full of anxiety on account of the failing health of his close and intimate friend Lord Carlisle, and went to see him at Palace Green, where he was trying "rest" treatment, and was encouraged to find him apparently better when he went again early in April. But the improvement was not maintained, for news came of his death on the 16th at the house of his daughter, Lady Cecilia Roberts, near Haslemere, whither he had been moved. It was so ardent a wish with Armstrong to be present at the funeral that it was thought best, in spite of the long journey, that no difficulty should be brought forward. He was asked to go to Naworth, but he decided to stay in the hotel at Carlisle, where were also Sir Philip Burne-Jones and Mr. Cobden-Sanderson. On the morning of April 20th they all went together to Naworth Castle, and Lady Carlisle specially sent for Armstrong to see her in her room. The funeral was on foot, though the place of burial, Lanercost Priory, was at some distance. A carriage, however, was provided for her father's old friend by Lady Mary Murray, and she and Lord Halifax went with him. He was greatly moved, and the family were all anxious about the effect on his own health. He returned to the hotel and travelled back to London the next day, Sir Philip Burne-Jones with him. Armstrong told his wife how much touched he had been by "Phil's great care of him," for he was feeling weak and tired. But he did not appear more exhausted than was to be expected when he reached home in the evening.

On Saturday, the 22nd, he got up as usual, and wrote some letters, but about one o'clock he complained of feeling unwell, and was helped to a sofa. The doctor was summoned, and was able to ease him somewhat with restoratives. His wife and their faithful servant of many years, Louisa Lawson, sat with him whilst he lay in a half-dozing state. At half-past four a palpable change came in his condition, and as the clock struck five he passed away, without recovering consciousness.

On April 26th he was laid in the same grave as his little son, after a service of dignified simplicity, attended by a very large number of friends.

The qualities which made his personality so attractive and lovable were his keen sympathies, his warm affections, his sincerity, his modesty, his able sagacity and his kindly wit. To his capacity of serving his friends, which has been exemplified in the course of this short memoir, he added the charm of a nature which preserved the zest of youth united to the wisdom of experience.

The bust of Armstrong, which is here reproduced, is the work of David McGill, formerly a student of the National Art Training School. It was exhibited in the Royal Academy in 1904, and its value as a work of art is enhanced by the fact of its excellence as a portrait.

It has been presented to the Victoria and Albert Museum by the sculptor, and the black

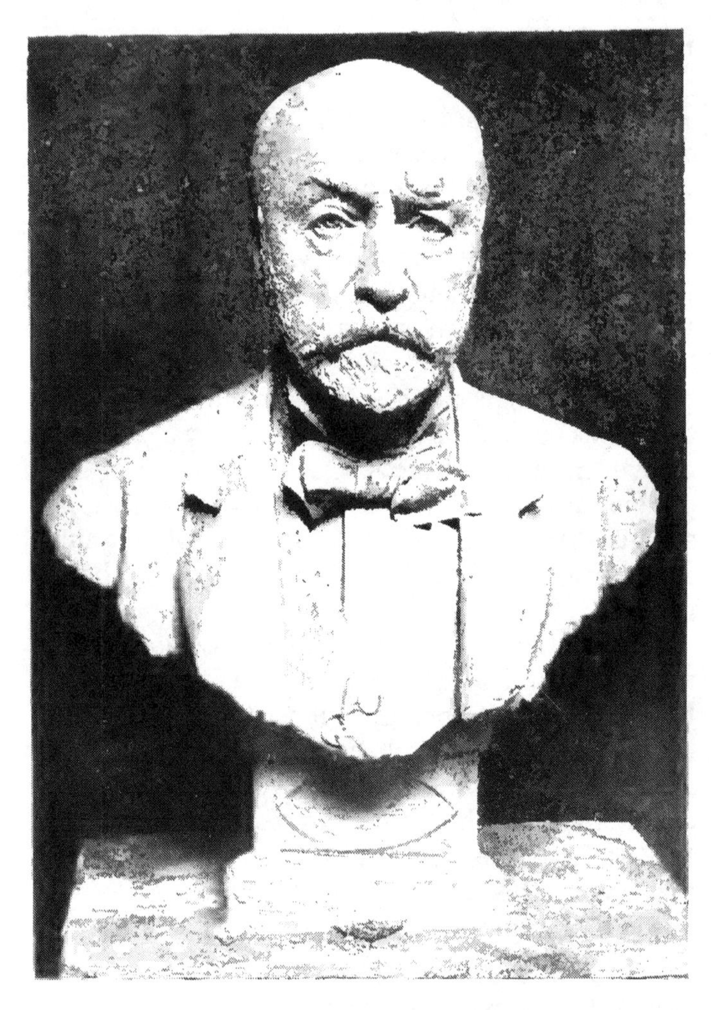

Bust modelled by David McGill in 1904
Afterwards cast in Bronze and exhibited at the Royal Academy

marble pedestal on which it rests is the gift of other personal friends. It bears the following inscription:

THOMAS ARMSTRONG C.B.
BORN 1833 DIED 1911
DIRECTOR FOR ART 1881-1898
PRESENTED BY FRIENDS IN
RECOGNITION OF HIS WORK AS
AN ARTIST IN APPRECIATION
OF HIS SERVICES TO EDUCATION
IN ART AND IN REMEMBRANCE
OF THE HELP GIVEN BY HIM
TO OTHER WORKERS

The authorities of the Museum are placing it by the side of the door of the library, amongst the memorials of others who, like Armstrong himself, worked with zeal to make the Museum an important factor in the industrial art education of the nation.

REMINISCENCES OF
DU MAURIER

REMINISCENCES OF DU MAURIER

THESE notes about the life I led in Paris more than fifty years ago have been made by me from time to time, and go back to my first acquaintance with du Maurier and others who became my life-long friends. I believed that the great popularity of *Trilby* had aroused curiosity with regard to the real life from which material was taken for the mise-en-scène of the story.

There seemed to be an idea abroad that all the characters in the story were drawn from life, and this belief was confirmed by the excellent portrait of my friend Lamont as the Laird. I thought that someday, that elusive someday, the reliance on which swallows up so many good intentions, I might put my notes into shape, and that they might interest those who cared for du Maurier and his work with pen and pencil. At no time could I have done this with vivacity and literary skill enough, but, backed up by reproductions of old drawings made some fifty years ago which I had carefully preserved, it seemed possible that my written matter might be made passable.

When du Maurier died, and again when I lost my dear friend Lamont, there were periods of emotion when my recollections of our early life together were very vivid; and so it was, but in a slighter degree, when Whistler followed the other two. If the work was to be done, it should have been taken in hand on one of these occasions. I am very old now, and scarcely equal to the corvée of splicing together my scrappy records and putting them into proper sequence.

Although my memory may have been failing somewhat of late, as happens to most people of my age, I am pretty confident that my record can be counted on for accuracy as far as it goes.

It is more than half a century ago, and much water has flowed under the Pont des Arts since we foregathered in the Quartier Latin as art students—"rapins," as they used to be called. I and the President of the Royal Academy are now (1909) the only survivors of the "Paris gang." Rowley, the original of Taffy, died in 1908, a splendidly handsome old man, surrounded by numerous progeny, sons and daughters and grandchildren, who have more or less inherited his fine physique; he was very proud of them. He lived on the Dee near Hawarden, where he owned collieries, and was a neighbour and friend of Mr. Gladstone.

Lamont and I, at the time of the high tide of *Trilby's* success, used to threaten du Maurier that we would give him away by writing "la verité vraie" about the events described in his story, unless he made it worth our while to be mum. Lamont's grievance arose from the ridiculous figure he made with his broken French in the book, and mine from being left out of it altogether.

I have always felt that the glorification of the clothing we wore, as shown in the illustrations, was something of a fraud—a pious fraud, perhaps—for did ever anybody see, south of the Seine, such faultless trousers, to say nothing of the well-cut coats, as those in which du Maurier dresses his heroes? They are sartorially on an entirely different plane from the clothes we did wear, for although we were not ragged or dirty, we did wear trousers which bagged at the knees. It is true that du Maurier brought with him from London some garments with the "vrai chic Anglais" about them, and among them was a Noah's ark coat (Does anybody remember the Noah's ark coat?), which filled me with envy and covetousness, so much so that it became mine by purchase or swap. The effect of it on his square shoulders was lost when I came to wear it, but I did fancy myself when I went to the other side of the river in it.

Before the coming together of our confraternity, known for a time in London after our return to England as the "Paris gang," I had had two years of Paris life, from 1853 to 1855. During that time I was working at an atelier under the direction of Ary Scheffer, then a painter of great renown, whose pictures fetched the highest prices known in those days for modern work; for instance, he had 15,000 francs, or £600, for the portrait of Lord Dufferin painted in 1854. I also copied pictures in the Luxembourg Gallery, and my friend Henry Morris, an able painter in the methods then in vogue in Belgium, was very kind to me when I was working there. He often came and helped me when I was copying Rosa Bonheur's *Labourage Nivernais*, which between us we made very good; indeed, it was said to be as good as any copy ever made of that much-copied picture. It was a commission, but I bought it at Christie's some years ago, and it now hangs in my house. In the winter months I drew from the living model in the evenings at the Académie Suisse on the Quai des Orfèvres. This Académie had an interesting tradition lasting through the first half of last century. Almost all painters, from Monsieur Ingres downward, had worked there at one time or another. There was no professor or teacher, but the arrangements for drawing from the living model were as good as could be had in those days; and Suisse, a very shrewd old fellow, not above doing a bit of picture-dealing now and then, kept splendid discipline among the fifty or sixty rowdy "rapins." Nothing was allowed which might in any way obstruct work, not even smoking. The place was always crowded on winter evenings from seven to nine, and we were much huddled together. There was no painting in the evening class, and I never attended the morning classes.

Lamont went to these, and he said it was a common practice with some of the students to look into the Morgue every morning to see if there were any new bodies. It was only a few yards from Suisse's door. One day as he was going in he met an old woman, holding a little child by the hand, coming out, and she muttered,

"Quel dommage! il n'y a personne." That would have suited me, for the only time I entered the Morgue I took good care to make sure before going in that no bodies were there.

Suisse was an amusing old fellow, and it was said he had laid by a good bit of money, which he left, with the goodwill of the Académie, to a nephew. The old man had been a prisoner of war on Dartmoor, and he used to tell us about the making by the prisoners of ingenious toys, which were sold to the country people in the district, and of his intercourse with them. When he came back to France he became a model, and sat to many of the celebrated artists of that time. It used to be said that all figures in Delacroix's famous picture of Dante and Virgil on the Stygian Lake were painted from Suisse, and certainly all those wallowing in the water, including the female, were very like him. Indeed, it was maintained by some that the boat also was painted from Suisse.

Most painters of note during the first half of the nineteenth century had worked at this Académie, and Suisse kept up friendly relations with many of them. In my time there were men drawing in the evening classes who were already known by their exhibited works. I think this admirable custom of continuing as far as possible disciplinary practice never obtained much among English artists. Etty was a most notable exception, and his mastery as a painter was greatly due to his unceasing practice in painting studies from the living model.

Immediately after the opening of the first Paris International Exhibition in May, 1855, I went to Antwerp to work in the Royal Academy there, but I stayed only two months, and then returned to England to see my family and friends. I mention this because my experience at Antwerp led to du Maurier going there later. I remained at home about a year, and, for reasons which I forget, gave up the idea of returning to Antwerp, although living there was very cheap at the time and the instruction at the Academy gratuitous. I went back to Paris and took up my quarters again at the Hôtel Corneille in the Rue Corneille, by the side of the Odéon Theatre. I had lived there before while copying in the Luxembourg Gallery, but while I was in England great changes had been made in the house. It had been thoroughly swept and garnished, and, though reduced in size by about one half, it had been made into quite a decent sort of dwelling-place, very different from what it was when I knew it before. Then it had on each side of its porte cochère a café with billiard tables, and, at the further end of the court round which the house was built, a dining-room at which many of the locataires used to take their meals. For these and for their consommations in the café they got credit, much too easily given by the landlady, who before I left reaped the fruits of her easy-going management in bankruptcy. The bailiffs came into the house and took possession of everything, putting seals on all the doors. Those who were out and came home to find the way thus barred to their personal effects were in consternation, especially as we were told that these seals were sacrosanct and the penalty for breaking them would be terrible. Anyway, I broke into my room, and was none the worse for the act.

The Hôtel Corneille was a very large house, having, to the best of my recollection, about eighty "appartements," the inhabitants being nearly all students of law or medicine, and a noisy, rowdy crew they were, singing and shouting to their friends below from the open windows in warm weather. There was no charm of architecture or even of picturesque delapidation about the building, neither as seen from the street nor from the courtyard. It was dingy, mean-looking, and dirty, inside and out; but most of the men I have known (I never knew or heard of a female locataire) who studied in the Quartier Latin during the first half of the last century had lived in it, and everybody knew it. It was here I first met du Maurier and Lamont.

There were two young Cornishmen living in the house who were walking the Paris hospitals, and from passing the time of day at the porter's lodge I made acquaintance with them, and was asked to their rooms; I say rooms, for they had a sitting-room, a luxury most of us could not indulge in. They had known du Maurier in London a little, and I found him with them when I first went in the evening to see them. I think Lamont and one or two others were of the party. It is strange that my recollections of that first meeting with him should be so vivid, but I suppose his personality from the beginning attracted me. I can revive the picture of him in my mind's eye, sitting astride one of the dingy Utrecht velvet chairs, with his elbows on the back, pale almost to sallowness, square-shouldered, and very lean, with no hair on his face except a very slight moustache.

Little did I think that I was meeting a man with whom I should have unbroken affectionate relations for more than fifty years. He certainly was very attractive and sympathetic, and the other young fellows with whom I was living at that time felt much as I did, if not so strongly. We admired his coats with square shoulders and long skirts, after the fashion of the day, and we admired his voice and his singing, his power of drawing portraits and caricatures from memory, his strength and skill with his fists, but above all, we were attracted by his very sympathetic manner.

Some years ago, when *Trilby* was at the flood-tide of its popularity, I met at a dinner party a young novelist who has since then much bettered his growing reputation, and as we walked home together we talked about du Maurier, whose books, he said, impressed him with the conviction that if he had had the pleasure of knowing the writer, he could have told him all his secrets. I think this was very much what we all felt, and this certainty of finding sympathy was one of his greatest and most abiding charms. His personality was a very engaging one, and evoked confidence even in those who knew him very little. A strange instance of the effect he made on people is fresh in my memory. He and I were invited to dine at Greenwich with some Lancashire friends of mine. (How very good those Greenwich dinners at the Ship and the Trafalgar were about forty or fifty years ago!) We had a very jovial evening, good food, "cuit à point," and excellent drink, just enough and not too much of either. We were all on the best of terms with ourselves and the world as we made the railway journey back to London. Two of our north-country friends were usually very serious and sedate people of reserved nature, the Clerk of the Peace for Manchester and Jonathan Tong, the owner of a notable collection of modern paintings; both are long since dead. They were as merry as grigs, laughing all the way at du Maurier's lively talk, which was incessant. I don't remember what it was all about, but it could not have been altogether what people call smoking-room after-dinner men's talk, for there were in the compartment besides our party (and mark, it was in a first-class carriage, a luxurious conveyance to which neither of us was accustomed) an elderly couple, man and wife, who listened with great interest and amusement to the talk going on, suppressing their laughter as well as they could for the sake of good manners. They were eminently respectable in appearance and of the good bourgeois type. They did not speak at all to us nor much to one another during the journey, but the fifth member of our party, John Holker, afterwards Attorney-General and

Lord Justice of Appeal, told me the next day that the old gentleman had accosted him as we got out of the railway carriage at London Bridge, and had asked him if we could be persuaded to go with them to their house in Printing House Square and be entertained there for the rest of the evening. These two old people must have died long ago, and of our Greenwich dinner party I am the only survivor. The incident has always remained fresh in my memory through its serving as a remarkable illustration of du Maurier's engaging ways. He was extremely amusing that night, but it was difficult to account for the attraction he seemed to have had for that old staid-looking couple.

After our first meeting at the Hôtel Corneille I found frequent opportunities of seeing him, and I also made the acquaintance of Poynter.

My English friend Arthur Brandt, son of a doctor practising somewhere in the Azores, lived for a while in the Hôtel Corneille when I was there; he was walking the hospitals. One day a French friend of his came to him in urgent need of money, for he said he was frightfully "dans la dêche." He had come for aid to a person seldom overburdened with cash, but a ten-franc piece was available. They went downstairs from Brandt's room together, and, lo and behold, at the porte cochère there was a "voiture de remise" waiting for the young Frenchman. A "voiture de remise" did not ply for hire on the cab ranks, and had a higher tariff than those that did.

Brandt was amazed, and exclaimed: "Tu

es drôle de venir m'emprunter mes dix francs quand tu te promènes en voiture de remise." The answer was · "Que veux-tu que je fasse? Je n'ai pas de quoi m'acheter un parapluie!"

We all used to borrow money freely from one another in those days. When one had more than he needed he shared his superfluity with those who were temporarily hard up; but we were none of us real Bohemians, for we had those behind us in England who would have come to our help if we had been in dire necessity, and we never knew what anything like bad hunger was. The worst I can think of was having to live on "riz au lait," a sort of rice pudding, very cheap and filling, which we got at the crêmerie, and it was very seldom that we had to pawn things. The delight of getting hold of money from the Mont de Piété was for the moment very great, but we found that effects, like watches once put up the spout, were apt to remain there a very long time.

In the evening we all used to frequent a café in the Rue de Vaugirard, a little to the southward of the Odéon Theatre, and we took our meals at a crêmerie or sometimes at the little restaurant kept by Trin, whom we came to know much better afterwards The summer was waning, and I was not well, so I decided to go to Barbizon for a time and try my hand at landscape painting. In this way I lost sight of my new friends for a little, and did not see them again until I came back to Paris in October, crippled with rheumatism.

Of my work at Barbizon there is not much to say, but I may mention that I stayed at Vannier's inn, the other one, Ganne's, being thought more expensive. The quarters were not very comfortable, but when one is young one does not mind that so much.

Barbizon was then, to the eye of an untravelled Englishman, a mean and untidy-looking village; it had houses at intervals on both sides of one long street, many of them with dunghills in front of them. There were no very interesting artists staying at Vannier's, but they were pleasant companions when we sat over our pipes after dinner, and I cannot remember any painter of note lodging at Ganne's while I was in the village. Millet, Bodmer, and C. Jacques (who up to that time had painted pigs more than sheep, and was called locally "Cochon Jacques") had houses of their own. Bodmer was constantly seen about in the forest, but he was not socially inclined, and avoided acquaintance with other artists he met. Jean François Millet was the only one with whom I made acquaintance, when he came to spend his evenings at Vannier's with one of the locataires, a friend of his. At that time he was a burly, farmer-looking sort of man, with a pleasant face and sympathetic manners. He had even then a reputation among the more serious kind of artists. It was not until long afterwards that I knew anything of his work.

We generally got up about six, and each, furnished by Madame Vannier with a linen wallet holding lunch (bread and meat and cheese, with half a bottle of wine), went off into the different parts of the forest where our work lay.

It was about this time that the administration in charge of the Imperial forests took it into their heads to plant a very favourite painting-ground near to the village, called La Gorge d'Apremont, with sapins (fir-trees), where there had been before nothing but heather, gorse, and rough grass, broken here and there by rock of a beautiful cool colour, the effect of which was very good to paint. The little Noah's-ark-looking fir-trees of a raw and disagreeable green had lately been put in when I arrived, and they were beginning to make a disastrous change in the hitherto pleasing aspect of the valley. Of the artists who frequented the village, some of the more adventurous spirits on one or two occasions pulled up and cut down a great many of these firs, and this led to trouble. I do not remember if any of the malefactors were convicted and punished, but by threats of very severe measures the authorities prevailed. New trees were put in to replace those which had been destroyed, and unless they have been cut and used for fire-wood they should now be well grown, for they must be more than fifty years old.

Beyond the Gorge d'Apremont was a space of quite level and fine greensward called le Dortoir, on which stood some fine oaks, singly or in twos and threes. I think this of all the parts I saw of the forest of Fontainebleau is the one of which I have the most agreeable recollections, and it was often painted. The Bas Breau, also within easy reach of the village of Barbizon, and through which ran the high road, Le Pavé de Chailly, was perhaps the most interesting, as it was left for some distance on each side of the road in a state of virgin forest, and not cut down periodically like the rest when the timber became marketable, according to the custom of state forestry. The undergrowth was very thick and varied in foliage, and there were trees in all stages of growth. Those along the course of the Pavé de Chailly were remarkable for the great height at which the spreading of the branches began. I have never seen any like them in England, though trees of greater girth are common enough with us. They were oaks, and their stately trunks of a light silvery grey made a beautiful effect against the darkness of the dense wood behind them. It was in this part of the forest that Bodmer painted the winter-piece with deer, which is so well known in the Luxembourg Gallery.

I went about in the neighbourhood of the village when the weather was not too bad, sometimes painting in the plain, and sometimes hunting for lizards and the strange insects which are to be found in the sandy soil, and I had the company of an artist who had a house of his own in the village. He had a passion for catching vipers, which abound, and this once cost him dear, for he failed to take hold of the snake close enough to its head, and it was able to turn and bite his hand. It was during the hot weather, when snake poison is said to be most virulent, and the effects of the bite made themselves felt at once. He had to be brought back to his house in a cart, for there was no kind of carriage in Barbizon, and he told me he did not quite recover for some months. My work, such as it was, was in the less picturesque surroundings of the village. I did a painting of the front of Vannier's inn, a building ugly and almost squalid in appearance, with a dunghill before it, but glorified by the vine which grew over its front; for the foliage of a vine in October, you know, is enough to glorify the dullest and dingiest of backgrounds. My little picture had some geese in the foreground; it was the first I exhibited.

Perhaps I am writing far too much about Barbizon and my own doings there, but it may be of some interest to hear about the place as it was fifty years ago now it has become so famous.

There was no talk in those days about the Barbizon School. Very many painters went there, and generally stayed at Ganne's inn. In it there was an oak cupboard, the panels of which were painted by some of the most famous visitors, and this cupboard was, I heard, sold after Ganne's death for a large sum.

Millet, Jacques, and Bodmer were the three painters most closely associated with the village, where they dwelt, as I have said, in houses of their own; but none of them would be considered as a chef d'école, neither would Diaz, whose forest subjects, known as Dessous de Bois, mostly done in or about Fontainebleau, are among the best of his works.

The only thing I can remember to justify the expression Barbizon School is that D'Aligny, a well-known landscape-painter, went there with his pupils. It was said that he had his followers out and marshalled them in line, "alignement d'Aligny," in the early morning, when he would take out his watch and thus give the word of command: "Sortez vos brosses aux peupliers! Il est six heures et le jaune de chrôme rentre dans la nature." It was told of Couture that he had boastfully gone to Barbizon to show how a figure painter could do landscape, but he went away discomfited.

The countryfolk about Barbizon were not comely. The men were dressed as you see them in Millet's drawings, but Millet had a parti pris, and in his revolt against the prevalent picturesqueness of peasant costume in pictures he went to the opposite extreme. It may be remembered how stiff the cloaks of his shepherds are, and how the ugly trousers never seem to take the shape of the leg in the least. There was a story of a friend of Millet's who, having ordered a picture from him, stood over him while he was working on it, painting the clothes of a peasant. The friend pleaded for a little relaxation towards the picturesque, saying, "Voyons Millet, un pauvre petit pli, s'il vous plaît."

Barbizon is a place now much written about by English people, and indeed for many years frequented by English artists. Before my time hardly any Englishmen had been heard of there. The Armitages—Edward, afterwards R.A., a favourite pupil of Delaroche, whose *Hémicycle* in the Palais des Beaux Arts he helped to paint, and a brother of his known as Bill, pronounced Beel—were much talked of at Vannier's inn, where they had stayed frequently. There was at the head of my bed, in the room I first occupied, a large caricature of "Beel" done in coloured chalk on the wall, and in another bedroom one wall was covered with a painted composition of the Wild Huntsman by Edward.

It was a common practice among the artists frequenting the two inns to paint on the walls. In the dining-room, the only living room on the ground-floor at Vannier's, there were many small landscapes in oil-paint, but nothing remarkable enough to be remembered except a common house-fly, so skilfully done, with a cast shadow, as to deceive one even when one knew of its existence. I think such tricks were common at that time, for in the atelier when I was a pupil of Ary Scheffer a palette hanging from a nail was painted on a door, with its cast shadow rendered most truthfully, the nail from which the palette hung being a real, not a painted one. At Ganne's there were more and better paintings on the walls than at Vannier's, but the best artists there worked on the panels of the cupboard or "dressoir" which I have already mentioned. Old Ganne was shrewd enough to see that the work of Diaz and the rest might become valuable, and would be commercially more negociable if done on a piece of wooden furniture than on a wall.

The rains in that October were persistent,

and my joints got stiffer and stiffer, until I decided that I must go to Paris for medical advice. I thought I should be back in a few days, but when I saw my doctor he said: "My poor fellow, you have rheumatic fever, and I must send you to my 'maison de santé!'" Accordingly I was taken there the next day by my old friend Henry Morris, and it was none too soon, for I had to be carried from the cab to the bedroom allotted to me. Here I remained nine weeks, six of them in bed, and a weary time of suffering I had; but I was much beholden to my friends who came to see me and cheer me up.

Maisons de santé, or nursing homes as they are now called with us, were not nearly so common in Paris then as they are now. Those in existence were under the direction of famous doctors in large practice, who could keep them filled. This one had evidently been a gentleman's house of some importance. It stood back a little from the Rue de Lourcine, from which it was shut out by a high wall with large wooden gates, and in the courtyard were several big trees; at the back there was a long and narrow garden. The staple trade of the neighbourhood (the valley of the Bièvre to the south of the Gobelins factory, which used the much-prized Bièvre water for its dyeing processes) being leather, the odour of tan-yards filled the air in all directions. I never heard of foreigners penetrating into that quarter, except those who went to my maison de santé, which was under the direction of a man of world-wide fame.

I had the least costly accommodation the place could offer, a small bedroom, for which I was charged 300 francs (£12) a month, and as extras I had to pay for firewood (rather costly) and candles, also wine, but of this I was able to take very little. The famous physician who was the patron came twice a week, and another every other day, and, besides these, there was a young resident doctor. I have always thought I owed my life to the careful nursing I got at this place.

Henry Morris came often from his studio—of which more anon—in the Rue Notre Dame des Champs; Poynter, too, was very good in visiting me, though he was always very industrious and busy. Of Lamont I knew but little at that time.

I was treated in a very old-fashioned way, with much colchicum, and was bled and blistered and almost starved; for nothing in the way of food except the weakest of bouillon was given to me. Sometimes I felt so hungry that I begged my friends to bring me a little bread; but they never did. I suppose they thought the doctors knew what was best for me.

My friend Morris, of whom I had seen a good deal in 1853-4, was an Englishman who had studied in Belgium, but who had at this time been long resident in Paris, where he painted pictures, mostly scripture pieces, for people he knew in England. I learnt that he wanted to go home for a long spell, and that he would like to let his studio in the Rue Notre Dame des Champs while he was away. So it came into my head that perhaps I and some of my new friends might join at it, and whenever Poynter or any of the others came to sit by my bedside we talked of this plan, and it grew. It seemed a bold venture, though the rent was a very modest one, for then and afterwards we thought the place very large for our requirements. But how small it looked when, thirty years afterwards, I persuaded Madame Vinot, the concierge, to let me enter it again while the tenant was out!

This hope of taking a studio and the prospect of our having a dinner together at Christmas greatly helped me to bear my pains when I was at the very worst, and this was pretty bad. My neighbour in the next room told me after I got up that the doctors came to him one day after examining me and said I was hardly alive; but even at this critical time I discussed with the greatest interest the very serious question of cooking the turkey, whether it should be boiled or roasted. A boiled turkey would be more English, to be sure, but we wanted to have a "plat" more English even than a boiled turkey, and that was a boiled leg of mutton, a dish never heard of in France. I remember how the water came into my mouth as we discussed this toothsome English fare, for, as I have said, I was kept so short of food that I was nearly always hungry.

The recollection of the planning of the Christmas dinner is still very vivid, and I had two other impressions during my life in that maison de santé which stay by me firmly. One is of the pleasure I found in reading, at the time when my pains were most trying, Alexandre Dumas's

Reine Margot, a story which, beginning with the massacre of St. Bartholomew, has a sustained interest to the end. I am always grateful to that famous story-teller for the distraction and solace he gave me then. The other abiding recollection is connected with a voice, a beautiful boy's voice, which I used to hear every afternoon about the gloaming of those dim November days. The air was always the same, a kind of chant, and as the boy passed down the street each day at the same time, I thought he must be a choir-boy coming from, or going to some church service. I used to long for his coming, and though the pleasure of hearing him was very brief, the haunting effect was always with me, and comes back to me now after fifty years, like the refrain in *Pippa Passes*

As soon as I was well enough to leave the Rue de Lourcine I went back to my lodgings at the Hôtel du Mont Blanc in the Rue de Seine. Although I had undertaken not to go out in the winter after sunset I resumed my former life, and saw much of my friends who had been so good in coming to me during my captivity. I also went on with my copying in the Luxembourg Gallery.

Christmas was drawing near and our preparations for the feast had been carefully made. The leg of mutton with a Christmas turkey and a plum pudding were coming from London, and it was settled that the banquet should take place in Lamont's studio, which was in an old ramshackle building behind the Ecole de Médecine, already condemned for demolition by the city authorities. The staircase was narrow and decrepit, and the rooms were on the third storey and small. I may mention here that Lamont held on to this place until one night in January police officers came to say that everybody must clear out of the premises there and then, as their state had become too dangerous for habitation.

The concierge was a very fat, good-natured woman, who took much interest in the Christmas meal of the crazy English, which she had undertaken to cook. Among the neighbours there was merriment about the boiled leg of mutton—"Gigot bouilli, Dieu de Dieu ! did anybody ever hear of such a thing ! Il faut bien être Anglais pour en manger."

I have been reading the account of the Christmas dinner in *Trilby* lately. The box of provisions did not arrive from London until six o'clock, having been kept at the depôt until fetched by two of our party, on account of two bottles of whiskey contained in it. These were seized, but Lamont remembered having seen in the Rue de Rivoli a dealer in English spirits, so on their way home they called at his shop and replaced the two bottles which had been detained.

The dinner was not ready until nine o'clock. How we did enjoy it ! There was wine, but for the most part we drank English bottled beer with our food and whiskey and water afterwards —"Vrai chic Anglais." It must be borne in mind that English drinks in those days were uncommon and dear.

Being an invalid I retired to rest in Lamont's bed at 6 A.M., but the others stayed on longer. Du Maurier had to go to Passy, where he lived with his mother and sister, and he told us, when we met again, that he had had a nap in the Champ de Mars on his way home. Everybody had been merry for a long time, and at eight o'clock, when the party broke up, they were all very tired and sleepy. I heard them go, and to the best of my belief there was nobody much " over the line." The next afternoon Lamont and I got up at four o'clock, lighted a fire, grilled the legs of the turkey, and with the leavings of the feast we had a famous meal.

I think it was on the following New Year's Day that we took possession of the studio at 53, Rue Notre Dame des Champs, and we were very proud of our tenancy. Four of us shared it—du Maurier, Lamont, Poynter, and myself—and for a while we only went there in the daytime. But soon afterwards Lamont removed his furniture to it—there was not much—and a little later I gave up my room at the Hôtel du Mont Blanc and joined him. There was a bed in the studio which Lamont used, while I, being still accounted an invalid, selfishly slept in the bedroom until Lamont himself had an illness.

The big wooden gate, porte cochère, opened on to the street, and next to it on the left as you entered was the porter's lodge, where dwelt Vinot and his wife and their two boys. Then came an appartement occupied by two young people, brother and sister, about whose position we were much given to speculate. They were picturesque and interesting in appearance, and we used to think they were people who had come down in the world. The brother was attached to one of the great public libraries. During the time du Maurier was with us we never got beyond passing the time of day with them, as they stood about or sat on their doorstep when we were going out together in the evening. He admired the lady very much as being of a highly-bred appearance, and she certainly was very good looking, thin and tall, with a great deal of black hair and large dark eyes, and with very finely shaped feet such as one does not often see.

There was no suggestion of Trilby here, nor even in a girl who used to sit regularly to a sculptor (a Count) on the opposite side of the court. We never knew this sculptor, but we heard strange stories of his practice as an artist. It was said that he had built up a figure entirely from measurements taken from this girl. She was very friendly and I think the Count bored her, for she often came to call on us. She was generally sitting for the "altogether," but being a decent and self-respecting body she always slipped on her shift when she came across the courtyard to visit us.

Up the next staircase lived Anker, one of Gleyre's best pupils, whose skilful drawing and painting we admired very much. We thought there was a great future before him, but the pictures he exhibited in after years at the Paris Salon did not realise these expectations.

These people I remember very well, but I have no recollection of the other locataires. Later, when Rowley was living at the studio after I had left, there was a sculptor named Maître in the studio beneath it, and they made friends. Maître used to box with Rowley and took his punishment like a man, and they practised the "savate" together.

About and behind the old houses in our street were gardens, and the trees which grew in them overtopped the high walls of our courtyard and gave quite a country-like appearance to it.

Vinot and his wife were great characters, and they figure in *Trilby* largely, being for the most part faithfully depicted. In the play Madame Filippi's rendering of Madame Vinot was admirable.

At that time most of the houses in the neighbourhood were of two storeys, and the little shops at which we dealt were very small and homely. This is all changed now. I have been there to-day (12th March, 1906) and found that the site of No. 53 had long been covered with a large new building, and all the gardens have disappeared.

There were two stoves, for we found it very difficult to keep up sufficient heat in winter. In the summer we used to open the large side windows looking over the court into the adjoining gardens, and through these the neighbours could sometimes witness the strange doings of "les Engliches," boxing, fencing, perhaps even bathing.

Du Maurier and Poynter used to work at Gleyre's studio in the mornings while Lamont began a large picture—we thought it very large, about six feet long—illustrating Keats's Isabella and Lorenzo, the subject of an interesting early work of Millais. I don't remember what became of it. One of us in fencing ran a foil through it, and after I had left I believe that Maître made a great hole in the canvas in falling through it to a well-directed right-hander of Taffy's.

Very soon we hired a piano, and friends used to come to see us in the afternoon. We used to box and fence after four or five o'clock, and du Maurier would sing. It was not considered seemly to put aside our brushes for foils or boxing-gloves until after four, and when Joe Rowley came to us from the north side of the Seine, where he then lived, before we were ready for play, he used to take silent exercise by walking on tiptoe without shoes up and down the studio with a thirty-pound dumb-bell in each hand until we "knocked off." It is a good exercise.

The drawing called *Ye Societie of our Ladye in the Fieldes*—Notre Dame des Champs—represents the members of our confraternity. The man in bed on the upper left-hand corner is Lamont, "the Laird" of *Trilby*, known among us as Tammie, and the likeness was a good one when he wore side whiskers and shaved his chin, as I did. Next to him on the right is the Greek musician Sotiri, who used to come often to the studio and play his own compositions, and other things, on the piano. We were much impressed by the fact of his having composed an opera, though it had never been performed, and after

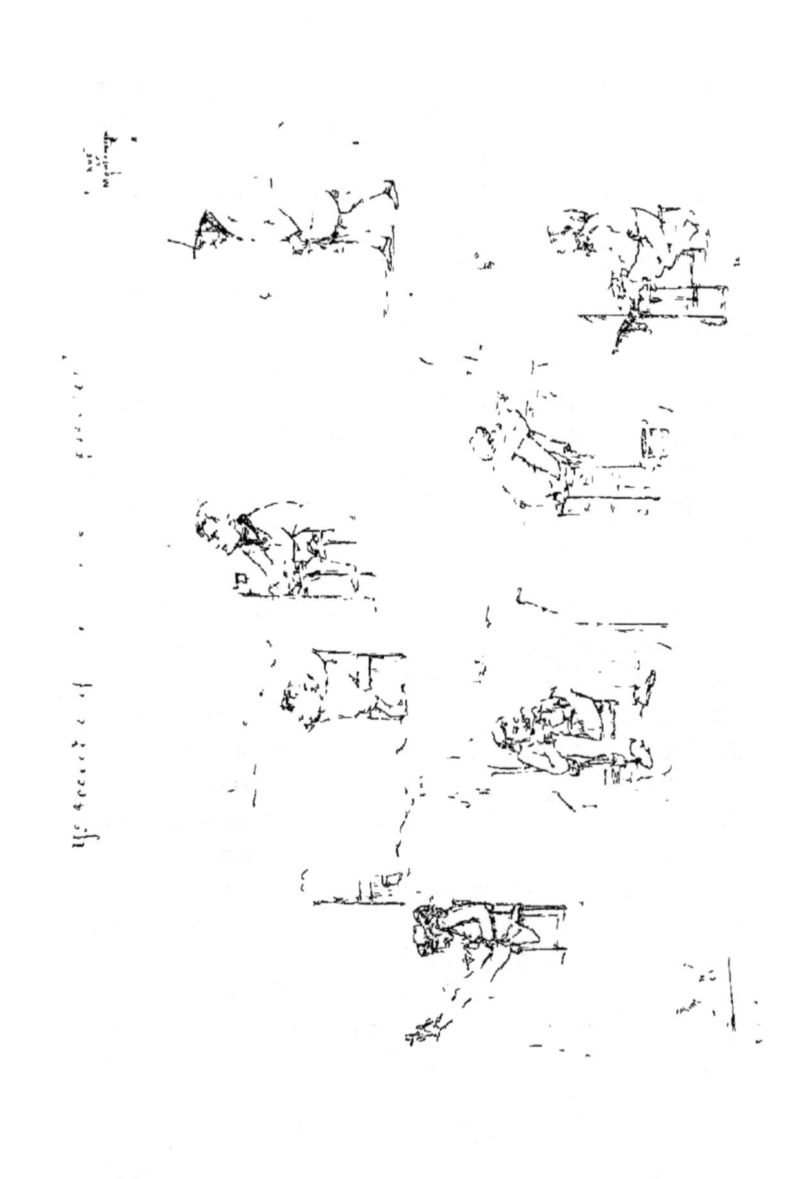

we left Paris we lost sight of him and never heard if he had any success in his profession. The figure to the right of Sotiri was meant for me when I was still much reduced by my long spell of rheumatic fever. Below me is Poynter, who was always a Nazarite, having worn his beard since it first began to grow. He was a worker who had been well and systematically trained, and we all believed in his eventual success; but he did spend a good deal of time at the piano, especially in singing airs from *Trovatore*, then in vogue; "Ah che la morte" was the favourite. He was some years younger than the others. Perhaps if he had been older he might have had a wholesome influence in making us work more steadily. Next to Poynter on the left is du Maurier, represented at an easel painting, a position in which he was rarely seen. Then, farther to the left, is Aleco Ionides colouring a pipe, his principal occupation at that time, though I believe he had been sent to Paris for serious study of some kind, not that of art. He is mentioned in one of du Maurier's books, and was afterwards Greek Consul-General in London and had a good collection of works of art. He came of a family by whom the members of our confraternity were received with the greatest kindness and unvarying hospitality after we came to settle in London. On the extreme left is Whistler; but this is not a very good likeness of him, though his curly black locks were worn longer than they were when he came to England. In fact they were what one might call ringlets, as represented in the drawing, in which, however, the hat is hardly of the shape he affected. He did not then separate and keep together the hairs of his white lock.

Some tenant before Morris took the studio had put up a trapeze and a pair of ropes with iron rings at the ends, suspended from a beam. They are seen in the drawing of *Cooking the Dinner*. This sketch was sent to me by du Maurier in a letter after he had gone to Antwerp. The representation of the studio, as far as it goes, is accurate, with the trapeze and ropes, and the confusion of foils, paint-box, and rubbish on the floor, besides a broom which I had been painting in my little Barbizon picture. In the middle stands du Maurier, who had been out buying victuals. He has the bread over his shoulder, and a litre bottle of wine in his pocket. This caricature likeness of him I have always thought very good, though the face is somewhat too juvenile. Lamont is cooking the chops in a frying-pan, which fitted into the top of our stove. His face is not so good as mine and du Maurier's. I am supposed to be waiting for the potatoes to peel, and am holding out my hand for them. He has forgotten to buy them, and in a dialogue written on the back there are or were some ugly swear words.

We did not go through this corvée of cooking every day, for we generally went out to dine at the little restaurant behind the Odéon Theatre kept by Trin, whom I have already mentioned. He was a little, black-visaged, bullet-headed

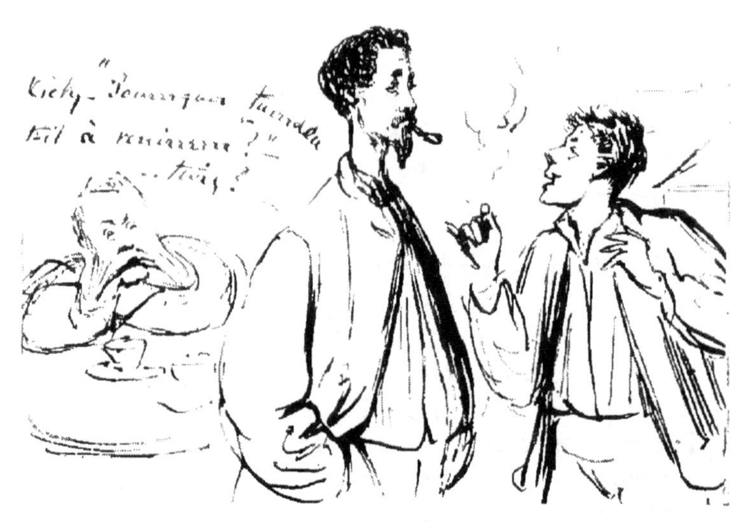

T. R. Lamont   Charles Keene   du Maurier

Pen and Ink Sketch by du Maurier

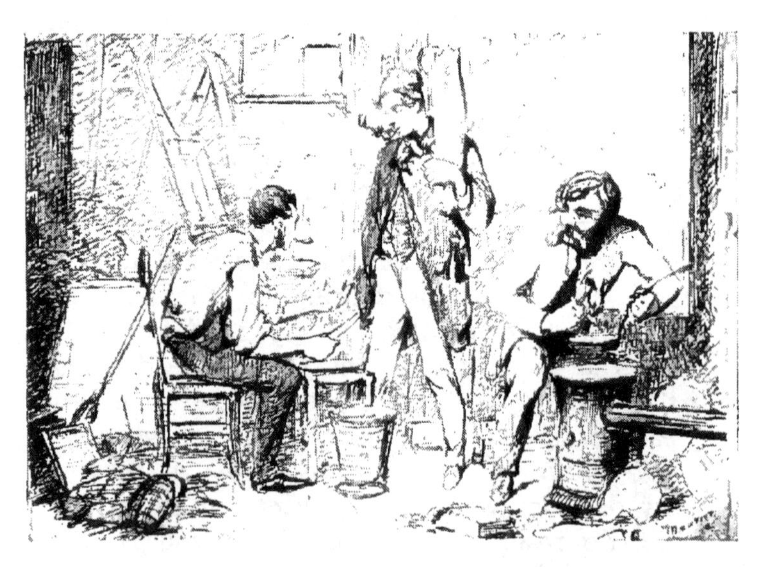

Pen and Ink Sketch by du Maurier

"Cooking the Dinner in the Studio"

fellow and he liked us, for he put up with our noisy misbehaviour with wonderful patience, and there were times when we were very trying. I went to see him once after the siege of Paris, and was greeted with effusion. He enquired most affectionately for du Maurier and Lamont, and wanted to treat me to champagne.

When we cooked our own dinner its material, though simpler, was of much better quality and much more expensive than anything we got at Trin's. We used to go to the butcher over the way and make him cut thick loin chops, and besides potatoes, which we fried (not very successfully), we had the best of salads, also in the season large melons. Our usual tipple was " vin à seize," that is, at sixteen sous a litre, or 3*d.* a quart, but when a guest turned up we indulged in " vin cacheté " at a franc a bottle.

When Marcel in the *Vie de Bohême* invited a man likely to buy his picture to dine with the " cénacle," did they not buy red, blue, and green sealing-wax with which they ennobled the common wine bought by the litre ?

We went out to buy the victuals, and carried them home ourselves in the clothes we wore while working. My own, for instance, were a flannel shirt and wide trousers of coutil, such as soldiers wore then, and an old straw hat of which a donkey had eaten part of the brim.

When Willie O'Connor, a friend and fellow-student of Poynter's in London and afterwards a very dear friend of all of us, came to Paris to study at Gleyre's he was got up to the nines, and his clothes would have borne comparison with those depicted in *Trilby* on the persons of Taffy and Little Billee. The first time he came to see us he had good well-fitting light-coloured kid gloves. He was asked to stay and dine with us, and I took a malicious pleasure in making him accompany me to the butcher's and carry home the chops in a piece of newspaper, and also the salad. This quite new experience was got through cheerfully and gracefully. We did enjoy those dinners of our own cooking, and we never had to go through the drudgery of washing up. That was always done by Madame Vinot.

On Saturday evening we generally made a descent into the middle of Paris and treated ourselves to British food and drink at a little place of no account in the Rue Royale (a much smaller place than Weber's, a few doors off), where the roast-beef and mutton, the boiled potatoes, and the beer and gin, were excellent and cheap. It was mostly frequented by people in some way or other connected with horseflesh, swell grooms, or men about horse-dealers' stables.

Here we had very jovial evenings, proud of our country's drinks. We were at that time like those wearing dog collars, about whom the old riddle was made, "Pourquoi porte-t-il des faux cols ? Parce qu'il est fier d'étrangler (d'être Anglais)."

One evening when we were very merry we took away from our little pub a sort of sign hanging on the wall with "Mince Pies" on it in large letters. Lamont took this (it was about three feet long) into the swell confectioner's shop for many years at the corner of the Rue de Rivoli and the Rue Castiglione, and, holding it out, said in English :

" Have you any of these ? "

" Mais certainement, Monsieur," was the reply, so he had to buy two or three, and with them and the sign in front of him he sat down on the edge of the pavement in the Rue de Rivoli and made believe to sell them, having engaged a street harper who was near at hand to play beside him. In those days the sergents de ville did not stand much nonsense, so we had to make him come away as quickly as possible.

On these Saturday excursions into mid-Paris we made our way by the Place St. Sulpice, where there used to be a huge wild-boar that was a joy to see. He was kept in a sty in a carrier's yard and could easily be seen from the square. We took the Rue du Bac in returning, and generally sang as we walked along in step, *En revenant de Barbizon.*

En revenant de Barbizon,
Zon zon zainé zon zon,
J'ai rencontré Mam'zelle Suzon,
Zon zon zainé zon zon.

Refrain :—

J'aime l'oignon frit a l'huile,
J'aime oignon quand il est bon.
Au pas, Camarades, au pas !
Zing tra la la, &c., &c., &c.

Or—

J'ai du bon tabac dans ma tabatière,
Dans ma tabatière j'en ai du bon et bien râpé.
J'ai du bon tabac,
Tu n'en auras pas.

I wonder why this rubbish has remained so fresh in my memory. Would that I could have retained useful knowledge half as well, for instance the dates of the kings of England or the allegations in Paley's *Evidences.*

Sometimes when the English gin had been mixed with very hot water we sang the Marseillaise. It is many years ago now, and the pleasure we had, or thought we had, in doing something of which the agent de police disapproved is no longer possible. Perhaps young fellows have hit upon something else which is forbidden to replace it.

We always made a point of passing by a picture dealer's shop in the Rue du Bac where good things were often shown in the windows. Sometimes we strayed as far as the Rue Lafitte, then, as now, a favourite street with the dealers. Du Maurier's fondness for those parts of old Paris lying south of the river and eastwards of the Rue du Bac comes out in many parts of his books. I too have the same kind of affection for them, and I have hardly ever been n Paris during the last fifty years without taking a ramble among the old streets between the Sorbonne and the Rue du Bac.

The Parisian students of those days who during the period of their pupilage had to make the wherewithal to live used to work at church pictures known as "Chemins de la Croix," generally of a common and cheap description. There was hardly any church in France without the set of seven representations of the events of the Passion, and at shops in the Rue Bonaparte and the Rue des Saints Pères canvases were kept in stock with the outlines of the compositions ready printed on them. These were supplied to the young artist wanting work, and he had to learn by practice a rapid method of colouring them with oil paint in order to make anything by this kind of job. There was a man named Cariage—who afterwards painted *Le Bilboquet*, a picture which made a sensation at the Salon—a clever pupil of Gleyre's, of whom it was said he could paint one in a day. The canvases, as far as I can remember, were nearly six feet in the longer dimension, and the price paid for each was seven francs; but this performance of Cariage was quite exceptional, and only to be achieved after long practice. The older or more experienced hands did not go in for refinements of delicate modelling and gradations of light and shade, but mixed two tints of colour, one for light and the other for shadow, helped with a black or dark brown outline.

The duration of pupilage in France was at that time far longer than it has been in this country. I refer to a time fifty years ago, when the painters whose technique has been taken as a model by the whole world (that is to say Europe and the United States) were getting their training.

It was not uncommon then to find men who had steadily persevered in such disciplinary work as modelling, drawing, and painting " bons-hommes " or " académies " (studies from the living model) day after day for seven or eight years.

At that time work in the ateliers began at six in the summer, and at eleven the seance was over and the class dispersed, many of them to do such work as I have described, or decorative painting of some kind to bring a little butter to their bread. The long continuance of this disciplinary work gave them a mastery in drawing and modelling the human figure such as our young people never have the chance of acquiring. It has been the habit of late among writers on art to deride it and say that the long training stamps out what they call " originality." Strange to say, the most successful teachers were those who had the least originality and whose paintings are for the most part quite uninteresting. Who cares anything for the works of Picot? Yet most of the brilliant and original painters of the latter half of the nineteenth century were trained by him. What could be more stodgy than the works of Heim and Drolling? Delacroix was a pupil of Guerin, but not long enough, and another great innovator, Decamps, was a pupil of Drolling. These men knew their trade and taught that which can be taught.

I remember a story told quite recently by one of the best and most accomplished of our own younger painters, one who is indeed a master in such painting as can be taught in a school.

He was inspecting or visiting a class drawing from the living model, and on pointing out to one of the students, a girl, the faults in her figure, said, "Don't you see that this arm is much too thick here and too thin there, and that you have not expressed the elbow joint at all? You must try to make it more like the model." "Oh," she replied, "then where does my personality come in?" This comes of the sort of pestilent teaching encouraged by many writers on art. They try even to vitiate the little wholesome drawing which can be taught in elementary schools by promoting the theory that the children must be taught to be "original."

When I was not copying at the Luxembourg I was working on two little pictures I had almost finished before my disastrous retreat from Barbizon.

About this time du Maurier did a little painting of Osbaldiston and Di Vernon. I took this home with me to England and sold it for a "fiver" to a friend, Mr. (now Sir) Edward Green, who had been brought to the studio in the Rue Notre Dame des Champs by Taffy, and whose friendship I have enjoyed up to the present time of writing. This little work is very interesting from the fact that the five pound note I was able to send him at Malines in payment for it was the first money du Maurier ever earned by artistic work. It is a good composition, and it is interesting to his friends as the only existing oil-painting by him, except a portrait of himself, done long afterwards in London, which shows very much better workmanship, but is unfinished.

Whistler took up etching in Paris in 1857, a process with which he was already familiar from some practice he had had while engaged on a government survey in the United States, but I don't think he told us this. He was very keen about it, and suggested that we should all get plates and try our hands. It was decided that each should choose his own subject, and that prints from the plates should be sent to some literary person in England and he should build up from them a story for publication to be called " Plawd," a word composed of the first letters of our names —Poynter, Lamont, Armstrong, Whistler, and du Maurier. We were very vague about the prospective writer of the text, who was spoken of as the " literary bloke."

Three of them were executed, Whistler's represented an interior. I don't remember it well, but think it was, in composition, something like Tassaert's well-known picture in the Luxembourg, a garret with female figures. Poynter's was in the style of the illustrations to Balzac's *Contes Drolatiques* by Doré, his best work, with which we were all much impressed at that time. It represented a French castle with many turrets dark against the sky, and from the upper part of it a beam or gallows projected with a skeleton dangling from it.

I cannot recollect what subjects Lamont and I chose, but I believe that the plates were never bitten, certainly mine was not. Du Maurier's plate has a personal interest, for in it he has represented himself with a guitar, earning his living as a street singer, which he thought he might be able to do if everything else failed. The miserably clad personages represented in the etching were, he said, "George Louis Palmella, Comte Busson du Maurier, with Madame la Comtesse and Monsieur le Vicomte." This title of Count was often a subject for banter among us. His grandfather had been made a Count by the Pope of those days, but his father never made any use of the title, and du Maurier always spoke of it with his tongue in his cheek. Sometimes one of us would make him a bid for it, and I remember that a bottle of English gin, at that time a rare and precious liquor in Paris, was proposed as a suitable equivalent. But there were to be thrown in to boot the title deeds of a certain landed estate on the Mosquito shore which had been conceded to his father. These deeds and the Pope's patent of nobility were left, some years afterwards, at Malines in a box which was lost and never recovered, so it would have been better for him to have taken the bottle of gin. The copper-plate of this etching was lost with these family papers. To the best of my knowledge it was the only etching du Maurier ever did, and there are only two or three prints of it in existence.

Music was a powerful influence in du Maurier's life. He used to say that literature, painting, and sculpture evoked no emotion which could be compared for a moment with that felt by a sensitive person on hearing a beautiful and well-trained human voice or a well-played violin. This, however, is all better expressed by him in *Peter Ibbetson.*

His father had been much thought of as an amateur singer with a very fine voice, and his mother was a good musician, so the influence of his surroundings in early life made for ease in singing. And sing he did, to the great delight of his friends in the Rue Notre Dame des Champs, and of their friends, and afterwards of many other people in England. He spent much more time playing on our hired piano than he did before an easel. In one of his books there is an account of the hero going out street-singing with a guitar, and meeting with much pecuniary success. This was founded on fact, and happened when he was a student at University College, or when he was supposed to be in practice as an analytical chemist.

He also describes another adventure in which the hero is represented as moving a rough audience at a Thames-side " free and easy " by his singing of a sentimental song, I think it was " My sister dear " from the English version of *Masaniello.* This was a great favourite with us rapins, and we also liked and called for airs from " tuney " old operas of Balfe, Bellini, and Donizetti. I believe he sang some of these songs with great success at the ordinary of the public-house at Rotherhithe when Whistler was working there.

When we made the acquaintance of the `reek musician Sotiri, mentioned as appearing in the Society of our Lady in the Fields, he used to sing to the maestro's accompaniment. We made a great deal of the writer of the opera which had never been performed, as none of us had ever before known a composer. There was nothing in him to suggest Svengali, for he was a mild-mannered sort of man, little given to assert his views about music, and he never showed any symptoms of being a mesmerist. The Laird, who had a sweet voice and a pretty musical taste, used to sing Scotch songs to us. Then and afterwards du Maurier often gave Thackeray's *Little Billee,* on which he had made musical variations.

But of all the songs in these early days I think the most popular was du Maurier's *Le Vin à Quatre Sous*—

Fi ! de ces vins d'Espagne,
Ils ne sont pas faits pour nous.
C'est le vin à quatre sous
Qui nous sert de Champagne—

and this was well known afterwards in London wherever he went. After he left Paris and went to study at the Antwerp Academy, where the dreadful and far-reaching failure of his sight from detachment of the retina was first noticed, he fell in with Felix Moscheles, who has written an interesting account of the life they led together. There was much music at Moscheles's rooms, where Brassin, a powerful pianist, was a frequent visitor.

When I was in Paris on my way to Italy in 1871 I went to see the old studio, and found in the immediate neighbourhood many marks of the German bombardment. Most of the shopkeepers we had dealt with were still living, and when Madame Vinot, the concierge's wife, went to tell them of my visit we had a sort of little meeting in the street, at which two friends of mine who were waiting for me in a carriage hard by were vastly amused.

Quesnel, the marchand de vin, came forward to meet me with so much warmth of gesture that I was afraid he would kiss me. His wife had become much stouter and more matronly, but she was still comely, and I shouldn't have minded being kissed by her; however she didn't offer. I think these good people all liked us, though they did think us a little crazy. Quesnel showed me where a German shell had come into his premises, and several of the buildings about bore marks of the firing.

Du Maurier has described in *Trilby* a visit made by his heroes to the old atelier. I think I saw it in 1889 when Madame Vinot, in the absence of the tenant, let me into it. I have already said it seemed very small, though we used to think it fine and large. There was no foot of Trilby or any other on the wall. I wonder how that fancy was developed; I suppose the fine feet of the dark lady I mentioned as our neighbour suggested it. The ropes and the trapeze were still hanging from the beam.

In 1860 du Maurier returned to England from Dusseldorf and places in Belgium, where he had been under treatment for his terribly impaired eyesight. Detachment of the retina which, while he was in Antwerp, had made one eye useless, appeared soon afterwards in the other, and was a source of terror to him to the end of his life. He lived first in Newman Street, and afterwards in Berners Street. I remember a house near the northern end of Newman Street in which he and Whistler joined in a room. It was long and narrow, with a window at one end looking out to the back, and about the middle of it a string was fixed across from wall to wall. Over this hung a piece of silk drapery about the size of two pocket handkerchiefs. This was supposed to separate the parlour from the bedroom. I have often heard du Maurier speak of the way in which Whistler kept him awake far into the morning hours when they lived together, telling of the wonderful adventures he had had during the day. He felt himself at that time greatly attracted to Whistler, and he was vastly impressed by his cleverness in many ways; but after a while this life à deux became impossible, for Jimmy was so very inconsiderate and exacting.

I happened to be at this place one day when du Maurier's uncle, a charming old gentleman who in early life had been in a crack cavalry regiment, came to see his nephew there. Hardly any kind of visitor could have had less sympathy with the Bohemian life he and Whistler were living then, but the Captain, who was good-looking and very well groomed, put on a good face and made believe that the quarters were much to his taste. N.B. There was more than one chair.

My visits to London about this time were not frequent or very long. I used to stay in Newman Street, and we all dined at a little eating-house in Castle Street, near Cavendish Square. It was a homely sort of place, frequented mostly by people who looked like gentlemen's servants. We were allowed to do pretty much as we liked, and the waiting was done by women with whom we were favourites. There came a time however when we felt we were getting up in the world, and might venture to a more "toney" and expensive place, a place to which one could give a French name, and call a restaurant. So Charles Keene was asked to prospect at Pamphilon's in Argyle Street. He was to find out whether the prices there were within our means, and also to report on the kind of people who were habitués, and to judge from their appearance if they would be too respectable to tolerate us. He gave a most satisfactory report, so we migrated from Castle Street to Argyle Street, and for many years afterwards some of us were always to be found there at dinner time. Besides the "Paris gang" some of Keene's Scotch friends used to dine there, and now and then Marks and Walker.

In those days (it is more than forty years ago) most eating-houses of this sort in London were closed on Sundays, and this was very inconvenient for young people like ourselves. Many of us were fortunate in having friends who were kind enough to ask us to dine with them on that day, but if we had no such invitations we had to resort to some more expensive place. About this time or soon afterwards the Arts Club was established in Tenterden Street, Hanover Square, and some of our friends took to dining there, or at a School of Cookery in Berners Street, which had a restaurant for the consumption of the material used for the lessons.

It was in a beautiful old house in the north-west corner of the square that the Club was then situated. The hall and staircase were of admirable proportions, and all the rooms on the first floor were sumptuously decorated. In two of them were painted ceilings, said to be the work of Angelica Kauffman, one of them a copy of Guido's *Aurora*, and there were three fine mantel-pieces of coloured marble, excellent in design and well executed. The house seems to have been remodelled lately for business purposes, and the club is now in less beautiful, but more convenient premises in Dover Street.

I have no distinct recollection of all the periodicals for which du Maurier drew. Work came to him slowly but increasingly. For a long time The Leisure Hour was a great stand-by, and for it he illustrated long serial stories. He took any work he could get in those days, gradually obtaining better prices. It was a great day when his work first got admission to Punch, for which he did many initial letters in a casual sort of way before he had commissions for any large drawings. I don't remember his having any other gagne-pain at this time, but others among our friends made money by designing and making cartoons for stained-glass windows.

When Once a Week was started du Maurier found a place among its artists. This paper was perhaps more important than any other in furthering the new movement in drawing on wood, which may be said to have begun in Moxon's illustrated edition of Tennyson. The advent of Frederick Walker was most important, and his development in its most interesting stages may be studied in the pages of Once a Week. His first appearance there was made in drawings illustrating a story about a diamond ring, and when he did them the influence of John Gilbert was still paramount; so much so indeed that any young fellow who wanted black-and-white work found it best to draw as far as possible in Gilbert's manner, to which the wood-engravers were accustomed. As one goes on turning over the pages of Once a Week one soon finds another story illustrated by Walker in which there is a marked change. This occurs especially in a drawing of a boy crossing a field by a diagonal path and stooping to pick up something. All artists were vastly interested in this talented young man, then little known, but afterwards so famous and popular.

Millais, who was one of the contributors to Moxon's Tennyson, did some of his best work for wood-engraving in this paper, but these drawings are not so well remembered as those made for Trollope's serial stories appearing in The Cornhill Magazine. I think Millais did good by joining the ranks of wood-draughtsmen, for his position was so strong that he could command not only the highest prices, but the methods by which the wood-engraver should cut the blocks that he drew. Leech used to grumble about his work not being well-rendered by Swain, the excellent engraver who did most of the Punch cuts, but it seemed to me that he was in this matter very unreasonable (though I did not dare tell him so). He made his drawings with lead pencil, and he seemed to expect that in facsimile engraving Swain should be able to give the soft edges of the grey lines. I don't remember whether Leech or Swain or both together hit upon the expedient of cutting a thin white line up the middle of a thick black one. Anyway it was a notable invention, and the advantage of it may easily be seen in Leech's Punch drawings for some time before his death. Young fellows who had to take what they could get and be thankful tried mostly to draw in a style which should be easy and inexpensive to cut. I used to hear much on this subject, and learnt that certain cross-hatchings gave lozenges which were anathema to the engraver and must be studiously avoided.

Charles Keene made a great and rather sudden move forward in the drawings he did for Charles Reade's serial story *A Good Fight,* published in Once a Week. His execution was admirable then and afterwards in its simplicity and its suitability for cutting. Sandys was, after Millais, the most highly paid of the artists who worked for this periodical, and something of his lordly ways and of his attitude towards the engraver of those days may be gathered by his remark to the editor, when he complained of his work having been ruined by the engraver: "If the small sum you give me for the drawings would serve as an inducement to the engraver to take more pains you had better hand it over to him." Few people seem to remember Sandys's most remarkable painting, the portrait of Mrs. Rose, a very comely old lady. She was the mother of Anderson Rose, an artistic solicitor well known to Whistler and other artists of that day.

Here I may say that having always in mind the excellence of the woodcuts in the early numbers of Once a Week I asked the proprietors of the periodical to search for the blocks, which were supposed to be stored in their cellars. They did so, and many of them were found, and from most of them prints were taken for the Art Library of what is now the Victoria and Albert Museum, where they can be seen by those who care to ask for them. Most illustrations, when a large circulation had to be provided for, were printed from electrotyped copies taken from the wood-block after it was cut, so the original block was not worn by frequent use.

I do not remember many of the drawings du Maurier did for this paper except those made to illustrate an account he wrote of his adventures at a Devonshire mine when he was seeking practice as an analytical chemist. Those who care to study his progress can do so in the pages of The Cornhill Magazine, and especially in Punch. It is no use writing about drawings or pictures unless you and your readers or audience have the things criticised before their eyes, for concerning works of pictorial and plastic art only clinical ocular demonstration can be of any use. It will be by inspection of the cuts in Punch that it can be seen how steadily he improved in execution and in the composition of his groups; and indeed towards his best period he seemed to show more sense of "envelopement," of putting his figures into the same atmosphere as their backgrounds or surroundings. I never knew how far he really cared for that supreme quality in Charles Keene's drawings and in the best of Whistler's painting; but if he did see and care I think he felt that too much was sacrificed to obtain it, too much of the human beauty, to which he was so keenly alive, in the figures.

He made drawings occasionally on Hampstead Heath when he had in hand an outdoor subject, but he found working in the open peculiarly trying to his sight, and therefore could not follow his inclination in this matter.

Leech used to carry little books in his pocket, and when out walking if he saw anything he fancied—a post and rails, a bit of fence, or the line of a distant cliff—he stopped to make a pencil note of it for use. There were piles of these little sketch-books when he died.

To du Maurier the shapes of a human figure as he knew them to be were of supreme importance, without much consideration of accidental illumination, and in his art as a draughtsman he cared only for the expression of this beauty. Herein he was a master, for who has ever depicted so charmingly the beauty of girls or children? They were legion and never quite alike, but mostly tall and stately. Sometimes he drew beautiful old ladies and noble-looking old men. When he had reached his best time he knew how to leave out touches in his little faces which were not essential to their charm. I never knew anybody who could be so helpful as he was in suggesting slight changes in the details of faces to make for beauty. He was of great service in this way to his friends.

He created a type, as it is the fashion to say nowadays, and nobody, to the best of my belief, has ever drawn so many lovely young women and children. Taste may return to high foreheads and sloping shoulders and the rabbit mouths of the Books of Beauty, but I think the best of the du Maurier young women will last. His imitators have so far not added anything to the charm of his type or improved on what he evolved. He was always studying faces, for which he had a wonderful memory, and he used to take pleasure in showing how the profile of the Venus of Milo's face cou'd be altered by taking away a little from the root of the nose in front of the eye. This he did by putting a bit of paper, cut for the purpose, over the part of the photograph which he desired to remove. This alteration had a tendency to give a more lively—though perhaps a less divine—expression to the face. It was however in his treatment of the tip of the nose that he made his girls so attractive. There was something of an upward tilt generally, and the heaviness one finds in the so-called antique noses was avoided, it may be at the cost of a little dignity. But there are no antique noses that I know of, except that of the Hermes of Olympia; even the Venus of Milo has had the extreme tip restored, and how much difference may not be made by altering that! I am of course thinking only of marble statues, in which the material lends itself to mutilation. There are some of bronze where the original shape has been preserved, as, for instance, the seated Mercury from Herculaneum in the Naples Museum.

As I am by way of dealing rather technically with du Maurier's work I may as well record his methods in preparing his drawings for Punch.

In the very early days he, like the rest of those I knew who drew on wood for illustrations, used pencil. He and Keene used to discuss very often and very earnestly the best tool for their purpose, and for the actual drawings on the block they took to pens specially chosen for the purpose. Later they worked with brushes after the Japanese manner, and for a time at least they were careful to use Indian ink. Drawings done in this way had the advantage of offering a clean definite line to be cut up to by the facsimile engraver, and moreover it was possible to see as the work went on what the effect of the drawing would be when the cut was printed.

Du Maurier used to practise methods of execution about this time with pen and brush, and I remember his careful copy of a portion of one of Rethel's famous woodcuts, *Death the*

Friend, and also portions of Menzel's work in the life of Frederick the Great. This book, of which Charles Keene was the first among us to own a copy, impressed English draughtsmen on wood very much.

The preparatory studies of the figures for the Punch drawings were done from living models with pencil, and in course of time he executed them with great skill and apparent ease. A number of these pencil studies were recently acquired for the Art Library of the Victoria and Albert Museum, where they may be seen mounted in juxtaposition with reproductions of the woodcuts published in Punch, for which they were made. For these drawings, generally representing people of fashionable appearance, he used to employ models who could wear his clothes and his wife's, nice clean people who came to him twice a week. I knew one married couple who sat to him in this way for many years. In these preliminary pencil drawings there was no attempt to give the heads, the places and sizes of which were indicated only; but the clothes were carefully done. From such studies he drew the composition again with ink, adding heads to suit the characters of the subjects. These heads he would do from memory, never making a likeness which could be offensive to the person depicted. Sometimes friends, ladies, were asked to sit for him, but not often, as he had very desirable models close at hand in his daughters and grandchildren. Most people who remember the Punch pictures of the nineties will bear in mind the charming little boys who used to figure in them, for there was no lack of these grandchildren of all sizes from two families. Among them were those who suggested Peter Pan to Mr. Barrie.

In du Maurier's books, especially in *The Martian*, there are descriptions of school-boy life in France which accurately represent his own experience. In the earlier years of our acquaintance he used to express great dislike for French school-boys and their ways, both in class and in the playground, but I think his opinions were modified as he grew older. He always said that French boys had to work much harder than English ones, and that games were held to be of little importance among them. So far as I was able to judge his own education had been very thorough, and the things he had been taught he knew à fond. The school at Passy to which he went as a day boy when his family lived in that suburb of Paris was, I believe, the only one of which he had any experience in France.

After his removal to England he was a student at University College, where he attended the chemical course under Professor Williamson, one of his fellow-students there being our friend Sir Henry Roscoe, who survives, I am happy to say. I never heard him speak of any literary courses at this place. It was his father's intention that he should become an analytical chemist, and for a short time, between his leaving col ege and beginning to draw from the antique at the British Museum, he had an office where he was supposed to ply this profession. While he had this place of business one of his father's friends who was interested in a Devonshire mine, then claiming to produce gold (according to its samples) at so high a rate as to raise suspicion among the wary, engaged him to go down and watch for twenty-four hours everything which came from the mine, and the subsequent crushing of the ore. This he did, with the result that the yield of gold turned out to be no more than can fairly be looked for in many such mines; enough to raise false hopes, but not enough to render a good dividend. His mission was satisfactorily accomplished, and it was made clear that the previous returns had been falsified by the introduction of gold from elsewhere.

Years afterwards, when he was drawing for Once a Week, he wrote an account of this adventure and made the drawings I have mentioned to illustrate it. This, to the best of my belief, was the first publication of any writing of his. I think he had made earlier attempts; in fact I have found lately, among some old papers, a little narrative of a scene he witnessed in a café at Malines, while living there with his mother. I know that he tried to make something of our adventures in Paris, choosing as suitable subjects the Christmas dinner at Lamont's studio, and the ball at 53, Rue Notre Dame des Champs, but he could never satisfy himself with these.

At times when the outlook was dark, through fresh trouble in his eyes, I used to urge him to try his hand at writing, but I do not remember any attempt in prose beyond those I have mentioned. He took great pleasure in making verses, and some of these are well known to readers of Punch; many others, as verse-making quite as good as the best of these, were too intimately personal or too trivial for publication.

He told us that French school-boys did not have to make Latin verses as we did, but they were well trained in French prosody. He at least had been, and he seemed to be master of its complications.

I remember an evening we spent together at Simeon Solomon's studio in Howland Street, when the early French poets, Ronsard, Marot, and François Villon, were discussed by him and Rossetti with reference to the later prosody of Malherbe. I think du Maurier started the subject. It was a very memorable occasion, as it was the first time either of us had met Rossetti or Swinburne. This discussion led to an exhibition of the extraordinary memory of the latter. Burne-Jones, Stanhope, Madox-Brown, Boyce, Arthur Hughes, and others belonging to the "clique," were of the party, which must have been in 1865, seven years before Rossetti's manuscript poems were published, which in despair he had thrown into the coffin of his wife. A propos of Villon, Swinburne spoke of the admirable translation of *Les Neiges d'Antan*, and after asking Rossetti in vain to try and remember it, he himself recited it without hesitation as it is printed in the collection of Rossetti's poems. He afterwards repeated the

French original. It was said that Swinburne had seen and read the manuscript once only, and it must have been several years earlier, for Mrs. Rossetti had died in 1862. These recitations led to others from his manuscript poems, afterwards published in the *Poems and Ballads*, and we both came away very much impressed by what we had heard. It was something like a revelation to us. We both knew the *Atalanta in Calydon*, which had been already published, but in these other poems, as I say still in manuscript, there were rhythms and metres which were new to us, word music most melodious and fascinating. Neither of us could ever forget that evening.

From time to time du Maurier made verses, which, after appearing in Punch or The Cornhill Magazine, have been collected and published, but I do not know of any prose compositions until he had been some time at work on *Peter Ibbetson*. It was not natural that he should talk much to me about the important new venture, for I was not at all sympathetic. When there seemed to be little hope of his eyesight holding out long, I was always urging him to try writing, but about the time he began *Peter Ibbetson* his position as a draughtsman was assured, so it appeared to me that by devoting to new methods any of the spare time during which he thought it prudent to use his eyes, he might soon find himself obliged to give up some of the minute drawing he did for Punch.

He had practised water-colour painting a little, and had finished and sold at good prices several elaborate water-colour reproductions of cuts which had appeared in Punch. These were executed with considerable skill, but the compositions did not lend themselves to this elaborately wrought kind of picture, though admirable for their original purpose as black-and-white compositions in line, going hand in hand with clever and funny legends. He had not patience to make fresh designs composed without thought of book illustration or legend.

It was my belief that if he could have persevered he might have got a vogue for small portraits in water-colour, which would have been very profitable. He did such portraits of his daughters, which had great merit, and with practice he would very soon have improved on them. In the likeness he did of his great friend Canon Ainger he had a very difficult subject, too difficult for any one. I have always thought the little pen drawing he made of Frederick Locker (Locker-Lampson) one of the best things of the kind I have ever seen. It was a striking likeness, giving all the good points, and the attitude was characteristic; but then Locker was just as exceptionally favourable a subject for pictorial representation as the Canon was the reverse. It was, then, because I thought he was neglecting opportunities of success in a new kind of work, which would bring him more fame and considerable profit, if his sight grew worse, that I looked with a "mauvais œil" on the distraction of story-writing; for his energy, it was evident, to my regret, was being more and more directed into the channel of his new work.

It was natural therefore that he should not confide much in a person so little sympathetic. I think his Hampstead neighbours, Canon Ainger and Mr. Basil Champneys, knew more of his literary plans than I did or any of his old friends, but he did tell Lamont and me, now and then, something about the story he was composing.

When *Peter Ibbetson* appeared I liked the book very much, and that liking has gone on increasing, for I have read it again and again. Although it was in a way commercially a success I did not see how he could by these means secure as much remuneration as when working with pencil or paint-brush, and the cost in eyesight appeared to be no less, for his writing was very minute. *Peter Ibbetson* prepared the public for *Trilby*, and for that he was paid at a much higher rate.

Trilby was a much greater success from the first than *Peter Ibbetson*, and when the American boom reacted on Britain and the name of the book was in everybody's mouth, while the dramatized version was being played in London, and by several travelling companies in the provinces, the incomings were very great and far beyond anything du Maurier in his most sanguine moments ever looked for. He used to say that nobody was so much surprised at this success as he was, and what a comfort it was for him to know that he need no longer suffer as he used to do when a fresh spot appeared on his retina and called up fears that at any moment his work as a draughtsman might be at an end. This was very cheering to him and his family, and all his old friends rejoiced at the unexpected prosperity, to say nothing of the gratification of his having acquired fame in a new direction and of having given pleasure and amusement to vast numbers of English-speaking people.

REMINISCENCES OF
WHISTLER

REMINISCENCES OF WHISTLER.

In 1855 Whistler went from England to study in Paris. At that time, as I have written elsewhere, I was there amongst a set of painter friends, and it was this year our acquaintance with him began. He was travelling first-class, and at some station between Boulogne and Paris, as he walked about the platform smoking while the train was stopping, he met and got into conversation with a fine looking Irishman with a big black beard (full beards were rare in those days in the British Isles, being then worn only by the followers of Joanna Southcott). They foregathered, and Jimmy joined the Irishman in his third-class carriage, when he learnt something of the aims and intentions, so far as they had been formed, of his new acquaintance, John O'Leary.

They were both going to Paris, but neither had any information as to suitable lodgings there. Whistler, however, had the advantage of speaking French fluently through his early bringing up in Russia, but the Irishman knew no French. He was going to Paris to walk the hospitals.

They agreed to share rooms, and when the Paris station was reached Whistler explained to a cabman the kind of lodging they wanted, in the Quartier Latin and not far from the Odéon Theatre, and he replied, "Je connais ça," and drove them to the Hôtel Corneille.

He used to tell the story of this adventure with great gusto and with no ill-natured intention towards John O'Leary, though he did heighten the colour a good deal. He "throwed style" into the narrative, as Huck Finn said of Tom Sawyer, and made O'Leary speak with a brogue and exaggerated Irishisms which I never noticed. When they got to the hotel the luggage was left on the cab while Whistler went upstairs with the concierge to look at rooms. When two had been found which seemed suitable in price, and otherwise, he halloed down the well of the staircase for O'Leary to bring up the trunks. By and by he heard loud curses and howls, and looking down saw him sitting on a stair and bewailing an accident which had befallen a rickety wooden box tied up with rope. It had fallen and come to pieces, and sovereigns were rolling down the stairs, for John's money had been put in loose among his clothes. He cried out "Ah well, if it 's been laking like that all the way along it 's sorra a few of them 'll be left for me."

However, I believe they were all picked up and the two soon found themselves installed in their new lodgings, two bedrooms with a door of communication between them.

Whistler evidently took pleasure in teasing O'Leary and taking advantage of his ignorance of French, but no bad blood came of this, and I may say here that I believe the two kept up friendly relations until quite recent years. There was a story about a laundress which amused us very much. She had come early in the morning while they were both in bed, bringing their clean linen, but the full tale of John's was not there, a handkerchief was missing. Whistler from his own room asked the woman to be seated, and when she took a chair he told John, who did not understand a word of French, that she said there was nothing missing, that he was making a pretext for not paying, and she would not stir from his room until she got her money. He had told her that Monsieur would get up and find the money for her if she would wait a little while. But John was in a terrible fix, for his night clothing was of the scantiest—a "cutty sack" in fact—and as he was a shy and modest Irishman he could not screw up his courage to get out of bed and cross the room to the place where his trousers lay with money in the pockets. There was much swearing, but, with Whistler protesting that the woman could not be got rid of until she was paid, the rush to get the money had to be made. It was no doubt a sore trial to O'Leary, who thought the blanchisseuse would be embarrassed and shocked, but she had no feeling of that kind.

O'Leary had a strong Irish intonation, but he spoke English like the educated man he was. His pronunciation of French was most extraordinary, and there was no room for exaggeration in Whistler's imitation of it. He was "très matinal le soir," as an old landlady of mine used to say of me, a bad getter-up in the morning, even when no washerwoman was sitting by his bed to keep him under cover of the bedclothes.

In order to attend the clinique at the hospital, which he came to Paris to do, as he had not taken any qualifying medical degree before leaving Ireland, he went to live opposite the hospital of La Charité, after leaving the Hôtel Corneille, so as to be close at hand. At the end of three months' residence there, however, he had not once got into the wards at seven o'clock, the hour of the doctors' visit. He thought another hospital might bring him better luck, and he moved into a lodging-house opposite La Pitié; but the great difficulty could not be surmounted even there, so I was told, for all I have written about O'Leary was told me by Whistler and Lamont.

I have a most vivid recollection of my first sight of Whistler, as vivid almost as that of my first meeting with du Maurier, and no wonder, for his appearance, at all times remarkable, was on that occasion most startling, "mirabolant," as one used to say. I remember the exact spot at the corner of the Odéon Theatre where I first caught sight of him, and his image rises before me as I think of it. It was in the warm weather of August or September, and he was clothed entirely in white duck (quite clean too!), and on his head he wore a straw hat of an American shape not yet well known in Europe, very low in the crown and stiff in the brim, bound with a black ribbon with long ends hanging down behind. At that time, and long afterwards, the ringlets of his black curly hair were much longer than he wore them when he became well known in London, and the white hairs were not carefully gathered into one lock.

Lamont had made his acquaintance some time before I did; indeed, I think they lived for a time in the same house, for I know the Laird helped to rig him out for an evening party when most of Jimmy's good clothes had been put "up the spout." Thackeray was in Paris at that time with his family, and gave an evening party to which Whistler, who was known to them through the Hadens, was invited. It used to be told with great gusto how the garments necessary for evening dress were got together. There was great difficulty about shoes of proper quality, but this was surmounted by waiting until most of the inmates of the house had gone to bed, leaving their foot-gear outside their doors, and then Whistler looked round for the nicest patent leather shoes of his own size. He complained bitterly that his unconscious benefactor did not have his shoes of a better shape, but somehow he made shift with them. Of course the shoes were put back on his return from the party. It was not easy to get new gloves, and I cannot do justice to Whistler's account of the masterly manner in which he cajoled the young woman at the glove-shop into giving him credit. I daresay all this was going to "chercher midi à quatorze heures," and that somehow or other a suitable costume for this party might have been procured by simpler means, but in that case the traditions of Schaunard and Marcel in the *Vie de Bohême* would not have been followed, and

Whistler had arrived in Paris full of desire to live up to the traditions of Murger's book. Like Tom Sawyer he was a stickler for doing things according to the programme.

Although he was very friendly with us all after we were established at 53, Rue Notre Dame des Champs he was not a regular visitor, but had other friends who were less " bourgeois " than we were. I remember one who was dirty enough, and greasy enough, and witty enough, for the most advanced type of Bohemian in the revered book. Stories were current about this artist and his landlord very much like those about the removal of Schaunard from his lodgings and the incoming of Marcel, when splendid furniture was represented by painted screens, about the only furniture they had.

This friend of Whistler's had none except his bed and his paint-brushes, which his landlord could not legally seize, but he had drawn, and skilfully drawn, on the walls of his room in light and shade, with charcoal, most beautiful and valuable pieces of furniture. There was also a tale about his avenging himself on an old lady who lived in the same house on a lower floor and who had complained to the landlord of his wild doings. She had a bowl of goldfish, which she used to put out on the balcony of the first-floor appartement, and her enemy, it was said, though I never quite believed it, let down a line with a baited hook and caught them one after another. Then he fried them, and by skilfully letting them down again with the line loosely tied round them he managed to shake them back into the bowl.

I think Whistler was thinking of this man when he said he should get back his shirt, give up his "no-shirt" friends, and live decently for the future. This was immediately after a visit to London when he had been staying at his sister's, where he said he found it very agreeable and soothing to be able to ring the bell and tell the servant to bring him a brandy and soda without being called upon to pay for his consommation.

There were some very amusing passages at a later period, when he had a very pleasant place to live in, with his own furniture, and allowed some of the Bohemian gang to have the run of it while he went to stay in London. I remember that he was really disgusted and angry with the effects of their filthy habits when he came back to the place. They had used all the plates on both sides, but never had them washed. That was about the end of his association with the unwashed, as it was after he had begun to make money.

For a time Poynter and Whistler shared rooms, and afterwards when Poynter went to the Rue Jacob, where he lived for a considerable time, Whistler took up with a very nice little fellow called Aubert, who was employed in the Crédit Mobilier. His services there brought him a very exiguous salary, but he was always neatly dressed and looked very clean, and we all liked him.

When this partnership had been running a little while, the eyes of both were opened to the fact that the monthly allowance each of them had dwindled away to nothing long before the next pay-day came round; so they laid their heads together to evolve some economic system by which their finances should be put upon a better footing. And this is what they did. Pill-boxes of various sizes were procured from the druggist; there were a few large ones for the month's rent, for the crêmerie where they took their morning coffee, and for the pension where they had lunch and dinner. Perhaps there may have been another for the washerwoman, but there were thirty little ones, each containing the small sum set aside for daily incidental expenses, " menus plaisirs," such as drinks and tobacco. This system seemed very delicately contrived and balanced, Aubert being, you see, a bank clerk; and you will probably be surprised to hear that at the end of the first fortnight our friends found all the thirty little pill-boxes quite empty, and there was, moreover, nothing in the bigger ones. I don't think there is anything quite like that in Murger's book.

During the time I was working in the Luxembourg Gallery Whistler made copies of portions of two pictures, the nude figure of Angelica chained to the rock in Ingres's picture and a group in Couture's *Décadence des Romains.* The painting of the former was not a bit like that of Ingres, for it was done in a thin, transparent manner, with no impasto and hardly enough paint to cover the canvas, also the colour of it was warmer and richer than that of the original. When we reproached Jimmy with not putting more paint on, he replied that the price he was to be paid would not run to much more than good linseed oil, for he was to have only one hundred francs apiece for the copies. The order was given him by a whaling captain whose acquaintance he had picked up somehow. There were to be four pictures, and I believe the other two were chosen by his patron from the Louvre collection. I mention these copies because I never saw any other specimens of Whistler's painting while I was in Paris, and I do not know of any coming between them and *La Mère Gérard*, which was done after I had returned to England.

He had a strange habit of picking up acquaintances in cafés and other places. I cannot remember how he met the whaling captain who ordered the four copies, but I have a distinct recollection of his foregathering with an extraordinary Irishman at the well-known brasserie on the eastern side of the École de Médecine, at that time much frequented by Champfleury, Courbet, and disciples of the realist school. It was a dark, dingy place with wooden tables, but had a great renown for its excellent Strasbourg beer.

This man had been a long time in Paris and spoke French slang ("Français de carabin") remarkably well, though with a strong Irish accent or intonation. He was a medical student, not very young, but he had never been able to pass the examinations to qualify himself as a practitioner. Whistler came to see us one day and told how he had made a very interesting acquaintance, and certainly his account of what passed between them was amusing. The Irishman, after getting into speech with him, had explained that there were no examinations going on just then, and he came daily to the brasserie and was generally drunk about that time of day. When Jimmy asked him to call, so that the acquaintance might be improved, he repeated that he was generally drunk, and asked, " Will it make any difference to you if I come drunk ? " Then he described difficulties he had had some time earlier (this as an illustration of his habits) with a man on the staircase of a low place known as La Botte de Paille, and how he knocked him down and then jumped on him. The Irishman was a very big, powerful man, and being jumped on by him meant serious bodily discomfiture. A fellow-student told him soon after, " There is an interesting case at the hospital," and the Irishman told how he " went to see it, and whom should I find but my friend of the Botte de Paille ; so I says to him, ' What's this that's come to you at all, me poor man, entirely ? ' " All this was said in French ; mind you, I should like to hear the French version.

This account of the meeting at the brasserie, given with Whistler's best verve, interested us so much that some of us went to make the acquaintance of the new friend. The narrative proved accurate, the man was drunk and said he was, and he went over the same ground about his habits and doings ; but, dear me, how deadly dull it was ! My only object in trying to tell the story is to illustrate Jimmy's illuminating power. He did not tell us anything he had not heard or leave out anything important, but by putting the accent in the right place he made an interesting word picture, just as he could illuminate for us a bit of a Thames mud-bank at low water (and there was a mud-bank along the Thames in those days) with a barge lying on it and a stump or two, things we should have passed by without notice, left to ourselves.

We English were lost in amazement and eaten up with envy when we saw the use our American student-acquaintances made of their Minister Plenipotentiary. If one of us had got into a little trouble with the police he would have thought it madness to send off to the stately palace in the Rue du Faubourg St. Honoré, which we revered so much, to ask Lord Cowley to step down and speak a word in our favour to the commissaire. Whistler thought nothing of knocking up Judge Mason when he wanted the American Eagle to back him up. I cannot swear that the Minister came himself, though I think he did on one occasion, but at any rate he lost no time in sending a secretary or an attaché.

The story Whistler used to tell of one of his appearances before the beak was in his best vein. Let any one familiar with French consider how, as a Frenchman knowing no English, he would write from dictation the name of our friend "Ouislla," pronounced with different degrees of sibilancy and in a low voice. At last the commissaire was obliged to write something and make believe he had got it. Then he was led on a wild-goose chase in search of Jimmy's nationality, for it was not until many guesses had been made that he had to ask point-blank, "Mais enfin qu'êtes vous donc ?" when he got the information, "Je suis Américain." By this time the commissaire was in a fury, and began to chide him with, "Eh bien, Monsieur l'Américain," and so forth, Whistler priding himself on his insolent attitude as he lolled over the edge of the desk. When asked if he could give satisfactory reference to steady, responsible persons—none of his rowdy artist friends, mind—he replied, "Yes ; my Minister and my banker." The name of the latter was given and it was that of Rothschild, at whose bank in the Rue Lafitte Whistler told us that he, like the rest of us, had now and again changed circular notes ; this was the only business there had been between them. Luckily Rothschild was not summoned this time, and Jimmy was allowed to go free without the good word of Judge Mason or any of his staff ; but he had a good scolding from the commissaire. After all he had not done much to call for punishment ; he had seen two well-dressed women on the Boulevard being harshly treated by serjeants de ville, and would not go away when he was told to do so, but insisted on seeing all that was going on.

It was not only protection in the police courts we envied, or thought we did, and I don't remember any of our friends requiring such backing up, but we were piqued by the help our American acquaintances, whose social position was no better than ours, got from their Minister in the way of admission to public functions, such as receptions and balls at the Tuileries. They hired the necessary clothes, but I don't remember what kind of dress was obligatory at the French Court then.

It was from a medical student, a qualified practitioner in the United States, then walking the hospitals in Paris, that I heard most about these Court functions, and when I told him that none of us English would think of asking for the entrée to them he explained how an American citizen was not on the same plane as a British subject : " For," said he, " every American citizen enjoys the possibility of becoming President of the United States, and is thus on a footing of equality with the king of any European state." I took it lying down.

I have no reason to believe that Whistler was gifted with a good ear for music or a good voice, and I do not remember his taking part in any serious singing that went on in our studio in Paris. But he often amused us with his nigger songs, songs of the old times before slavery was abolished and plantation life underwent a great change. He used to take a stick or an umbrella and, holding it in his left hand like a banjo, twiddled on it with the finger and thumb of the right hand while he pattered grotesque rhymes founded on the supposed adventures of Scripture characters. These were said to be camp-meeting hymns, and perhaps they were originally to some extent, but they must have been amplified and made more grotesque by white folks. I remember hearing afterwards in England something of the same kind and always with the same refrain :—

> Takey off your coat, Boys,
> Rolley up your sleeve,
> For Jordan am a hard road to travel, I believe.

There was one word in Jimmy's version which had a strange fascination for me, "alagoolacorden." It came in this way :—

> Now Abraham had a knave,
> And Isaac had an alagoolacorden,
> And he bet him his old hat,
> And when he'd won dat
> He chucked him to the udder side of Jordan, I believe.

I am sure I can trust my memory for the sound of the word, which I have written phonetically as nearly as possible. It has been a comfort to me ever since, as was the word "Mesopotamia" to the old lady.

There was another famous ditty to a different tune, of which the following cosmogony is the only part I recollect :—

> De World was made in six days,
> And finished on de seventh,

According to de contract should have been
de eleventh ;
But de masons dey fell sick,
And de joiners wouldn't work,
And so dey thought de cheapest way
Was to fill it up wid dirt.

The refrain was :—

Walk in, walk in, walk in, say
Walk in de back parlour and hear de banjo play.

There are not many living of those who were in Paris with Whistler in 1856–7, but Professor Legros and Fantin Latour knew a good deal about his career a little later, at the time when they used to work together in Bonvin's studio, sometimes under Courbet's instruction.

The later quarrel with Legros was grievous and not to be made up, but with Fantin I think there was no open breach of friendly relations. I remember telling Whistler about my visit to Fantin's studio in Paris and how I found him and Madame Fantin painting together there. He said, "Ah, oui, la peinture à quatre mains. Je connais ça."

I believe Whistler learned a good deal from Fantin, who was a very able exponent of his views on art. I read an account of his life and work lately, and was astonished at not finding any mention of the admirable copies he used to make. He copied *The Marriage at Cana*, the immense picture by Veronese in the Louvre, many times and in different sizes ; one at least of these copies came to England. I remember, too, one of Titian's

Supper at Emmaus. These were much esteemed by artists, and for a time Fantin made his living by them.

I have always thought that Whistler learnt much from Courbet, who was a very skilful painter, and, I should think, a very good teacher. The first important recognition of Whistler's talent I ever heard of came from him when, after criticising the studies from living models that were being done at Bonvin's, he exclaimed, pointing to Whistler's little picture called *La Mère Gérard*, " Mais que voulez-vous que je vous dise ? ça y est—quoi ! "

Many people have heard the story, I expect, of how Whistler, after being away from Paris for some time, was walking with friends up the Rue de Vaugirard towards the place where the Mère Gérard used to sit selling violets under the grille of the Luxembourg Gardens. It was proposed that one of them should go on in front and tell her that he (Whistler) was dead. Jimmy was to go to the other side of the railing to hear what she would say. The listener did not hear any good of himself. The old woman could not easily be made to understand what they were telling her, so they explained that it was about the artist who had done her portait. " Eh bien, quoi ? " " Eh bien, il est mort." " Voila une fameuse canaille de moins," was her only remark. I have always felt grateful to Whistler for telling us this funny story against himself.

There is another I had from him of the same kind, in which the joke was perhaps more rankling.

It belongs to a later period. George Chapman, an artist of fine taste who died without doing much, was a very old friend of Whistler's, and I think they were at school together at Portishead near Bristol. They were going to visit at the same house in Scotland and were travelling in a Pullman car, for the days of prosperity had then been reached. To relieve the tedium of their long journey George improved the occasion by giving Whistler a lecture on his pretensions and lack of achievement, and so on. In the course of it he said, "My dear Jimmy, you know you have had un petit succès d'exécration." "Succès d'exécration" is to me amazing in its appropriateness, or was at the time, and I think Whistler envied his friend the joy of making the happy bon mot. He had as he thought a kind of revenge, for while the lecture was proceeding he was loosening a screw which held Chapman's iron rocker in position, and directly after the "Succès d'exécration" shot had been fired, the chair doubled up, and Chapman was on the floor.

The Art Treasures Exhibition held in Manchester in 1857 was a memorable event, and a visit Whistler made to it had no little influence on him. The winter exhibitions of the works of the Old Masters at the Royal Academy had not then been begun, but there had been one in the spring on a smaller and less important scale at the British Institution in Pall Mall. Many owners of fine collections of pictures were members of the society. During the winter months there was an exhibition of the works of living artists. It may be worth recording here that this body was dissolved after the establishment of winter exhibitions of paintings by Old Masters at the Royal Academy, and its funds were applied to the institution of scholarships for students in painting, sculpture, architecture, and engraving.

To return, however, to the Art Treasures Exhibition at Manchester, where among many of the finest paintings owned in this country and hardly known to the public were also to be seen works of decorative or applied art, such as was formed by the famous Soulages collection. This was afterwards bought for the Museum at South Kensington, perhaps the most important purchase ever made for it.

It was in the summer of 1857 that Whistler, who had heard of the fine pictures lent to the Exhibition, turned up at our studio one morning to tell us he much wanted to go to Manchester with "le petit Martin," a fellow-student at Gleyre's and a son of Henri Martin, the well-known historian, who was setting off in a few days. There was a little difficulty, however, as to ways and means, and he wanted to know if, in our opinion, it would be expedient for him to ask for a loan from M. Bergeron, a sort of connection of his, who was, I think, engineer of the Northern of France railway, and who had before acted as a Providence to him.

I enquired if he had repaid the eighty francs the gentleman had lent him not long ago. "Well, no," replied Jimmy, "I haven't, but I don't think he expected it. Anyway, I'll go to see him and explain, and I'll ask him if he thinks I ought to ask him to lend me this money for the Manchester journey." He got it, of course, and no wonder, for the ingenuity of the way of asking it deserved success.

It was that visit to Manchester, when he saw very fine specimens of the work of Velasquez, which began to bring about the appreciation of the Spanish painter, whom he afterwards, so to speak, took into partnership Before that time I think we had all learnt to admire his *Infanta Margaret* in the Louvre, but Velazquez was not much talked about in those days. According to the public taste, *The Immaculate Conception,* by Murillo, bought about 1857 from Marshal Soult's collection for the Louvre at the price of £23,000, was the most precious picture in the world. In 1857 *The Three Maries*, by Annibale Carracci, shown in the Manchester exhibition, from Castle Howard, was accounted the masterpiece of the world. How long will it be before Guido, the Carracci, and such like come to the top again in the sale room?

I never knew Ernest, one of Whistler's most intimate friends, with whom he made the tour in Germany. Their money ran short through the miscarriage of a letter, so they had to go on foot, and they did pencil portraits of the inhabitants of villages they passed through to pay their expenses, at first charging a thaler each for them, and at last in dire necessity having to do them for a groschen. The bellman was generally sent round to announce the arrival of two distinguished artists from Paris; I think some of the etchings in the first set of twelve were done during this walking tour The journey was made memorable to many of us by the inimitable way in which Whistler related their adventures. There never was such a raconteur, I verily believe. As for his story-telling at that time, you may say of it what Courbet said of the painting of *La Mère Gérard*. He gave one the most vivid impression of their wanderings. The account of his lying ill in the hospital in Paris was equally vivid, and for the most part this was very funny, but there were pathetic passages.

La Mère Gérard was the earliest exhibited picture by Whistler, and I think it was also the earliest original work in oil. He was supposed to be a student at Gleyre's atelier at this time, but he did not work much there or elsewhere. I have been told lately that a letter to Fantin is in existence in which Whistler expresses regret at not having been a pupil of Ingres. Perhaps he might have been more regular for a while in attendance at the atelier with the influence and prestige of Monsieur Ingres to bear on him, but I don't think he would.

There was something strange about the way in which this prestige was shown when students would nearly always speak of him as "Monsieur" Ingres, while the other eminent painters were Delacroix, Vernet, Scheffer, or Decamps, tout court. This sort of unconscious acknowledgment of merit or distinction came from young people who scoffed at him, called his paintings "croûtes," and were always ready to rebel against academic authority and side with revolutionaries like Delacroix and Decamps.

There was a pamphlet in circulation in those days, a skit or "charge," giving a sort of biography of Monsieur Ingres which began in this way: "Monsieur Ingres ayant comme enfant beaucoup de disposition pour la musique ses parents l'ont fait étudier la peinture." He was an enthusiastic amateur violinist, and it used to be said that he thought much more of his skill with this instrument than he did of his success as a painter. I got into the way of speaking of Monsieur Ingres like the rest, and I believe I do so to this day. I do not think I cared very much for his pictures, except for the splendid portrait of Bertin, which I knew through the fine engraving by Dupont.

Among the early etchings by Whistler, in the set of twelve, if I am not mistaken, there is one of a seated figure of a girl, with long hair hanging loose about her shoulders and with a basket in her lap. This was done from Héloïse, a girl-model well known in the Quartier. She was a remarkable person, not pretty in feature, and sallow in complexion, but with good eyes and a sympathetic sort of face. As this was long before the fashion came in for women and children to wear their hair hanging loose, and not in plaits down their backs, Héloïse attracted the notice of passers-by almost as much as Whistler did when he was wearing "more Americano," his summer suit of white duck, with the jaunty little flat-crowned Yankee hat. She used to go about bareheaded and carrying a little basket containing the crochet work she was in the habit of doing, and a volume of Alfred de Musset's poems. This little pose added to the interest excited by her flowing locks and her large eyes. She was a chatterbox, and at times regaled us with songs, rather spoken than sung, for she had not much voice or power of musical expression. She used to sing :—

Voulez vous savoir, savoir,
Comment les artistes aiment ?
Ils aiment si artistement,
Ils sont de si artistes gens.

Spoken :—

Qu'ils s'en vont tout en disant :
Voulez vous venir chez moi, Mademoiselle ?
Et je ferai votre portrait.

Refrain :—

Ramenez vos moutons, bergères,

Sung :—

Ramenez vos moutons des champs.

In later couplets the amatory peculiarities of soldiers, lawyers, doctors, and others were sung about. In this Héloïse were some slight suggestions for the character of Trilby, but only in the basket of work and in the book, and I know of no other female inhabitant of the Quartier Latin who had any of the characteristics of du Maurier's heroine.

I am very sorry and feel like an impostor, but really this Héloïse is as near as I can get to the original of Trilby.

When we were in Paris together none of us could with certainty guess at Whistler's age, but he must have been about thirty, or younger, for he varied very much, and sometimes looked quite old.

Once he mentioned his mother, and Lamont exclaimed, "Your mother? Who would have thought of you having a mother, Jimmy." "Yes, indeed, I have a mother, and a very pretty bit of colour she is, I can tell you," was the reply. And so she was when I knew her afterwards in Chelsea, much more ruddy than she is represented in the beautiful portrait now in the Luxembourg Gallery.

Whistler at his best, and when he was well groomed, made a very good appearance, although there was always too great a display of hair. He had a good chest and powerful arms, but he never took any part in our athletic exercises in the studio of the Rue Notre Dame des Champs, but would laugh at us and say, when we were boxing or lifting dumb-bells, "Why the devil can't you fellows get your concierge to do that sort of thing for you?" His turn for boxing came some years later, when he took lessons from a well-known "pug" whose place was behind the Quadrant in Regent Street; I forget his name. The results were disastrous, and were much regretted by all his real friends. Having acquired some skill with his fists, and being endowed by nature with pluck and muscular strength, he thought he must put into practice the training he had given himself, and in consequence proceeded to try what he could do without the gloves. Then came the period of "voies de fait." I think there may have been some excuse for his fight with the mason, but he was evidently on the look-out for somebody to have a row with. This was not unnatural or uncommon, for I have known of professors of the noble art telling their pupils that the time for glove sparring was over, and that further improvement could only come from using the bare fists. Two of his assaults had, I am sure, a great effect on his after life, so much odium fell on him in consequence.

He would go sometimes in the evening to box with our friend Nesfield the architect, at his chambers in Argyle Street, and one night he turned up there very late, and insisted on being let in for a bout with the gloves. Nesfield got up and admitted him, but he owed him a grudge for the disturbance, and he paid him out for it. Nesfield had not so long a reach as Jimmy, but he was very powerful, and at the end of the bout he sent his disturber away with his shirt covered with blood. He said Whistler took his punishment very well and cheerily.

I think it was at the time of Whistler's great success with his picture *At the Piano* in the Academy of 1860 that Aleco Ionides first heard of his being in London and sought him out to introduce him to his family. Du Maurier and I were then in Düsseldorf, but when we and other members of the "gang" came to London, we were all frequent guests of these kind Ionides, who then lived at Tulse Hill.

So far as I can recollect there were no other artists frequenting the Ionides's house when we appeared, but in Watts's early days he had been a great friend of the family, and had painted the portraits of many of them. These portraits were, for the most part, rather brown and low in tone, done in the careful and laborious manner now called "stodgy," which alone leads to that mastery with the brush for which Watts's later work was so remarkable.

The friendly intercourse thus begun with the Ionides family lasted many years, and the house at Holland Park, where the old people afterwards lived, was the favourite resort of many interesting artists besides those Aleco got to know in Paris, notably of Rossetti, Burne-Jones, William Morris, Legros, and Philip Webb.

Rossetti's first appearance at the Tulse Hill house was on one summer Sunday, when a cab-load—such a cab-load as was, perhaps, never seen except at an Irish funeral—set out from Chelsea: Whistler, Rossetti, du Maurier, Legros, Ridley, and myself were in or on it. It seems to me that there were others in that four-wheeler, Poynter perhaps, but I am not sure, and I want to be accurate. The occasion was a memorable one. Then for the first time was revealed to this artistic circle the beauty of two girls, relations or connections of the Ionides family, and daughters of the Consul-General for Greece in London, Mr. Spartali. We were all à genoux before them, and of course every one of us burned with a desire to try to paint them. Very shortly afterwards Whistler got the younger one, Miss Christine Spartali, to sit for his large painting, *La Princesse du Pays de la Porcelaine*, which for a long time hung in the Peacock Room at Mr. Leyland's house in Prince's Gate. The elder sister, well known afterwards as an artist, must have sat to several of these friends, but I never saw any representation of her in painting which gave any idea of her sweetness and stateliness. I still see remaining in her, after the lapse of all these years, much of the striking nobility of form and charm of colour before which we all bowed forty years ago. I remember her, as if it were yesterday, coming out on the lawn of her father's house on Clapham Common when there was a large garden party, and Swinburne, who was with us, saying, "She is so beautiful I feel as if I could sit down and cry." She wore a dress trimmed with little bunches of ribbon of various colours, like that in which Rossetti represented Lucretia in his water-colour drawing called *The Borgia Family*, one of the best of his works.

I think Whistler always knew how deep and sincere my admiration was for his best work, and how earnestly I looked forward to the development of his great gifts as a painter by his overcoming some of the difficulties confronting him through lack of sufficient disciplinary training.

I have thought sometimes that I might record my observations of his practice at the time I was very much under his influence, but without having the things to show no words I am master of would avail much. I may perhaps correct the impression, common among outsiders, that Whistler's pictures were done in a rapid and slap-dash manner. I have never seen or heard of any painter who took so much time in making up tints on his palette before applying them to the canvas, and he worked very slowly. When laid there with his sensitive touch they were not worked on, but other brushfuls were put alongside them in the same deliberate manner, and there they remained unless at the end of the day he decided that the piece of work could and should be better done; then he took off the wet paint with a palette knife and wiped the canvas clean with a rag. This was his practice when he was, to my mind, at his best.

I remember well having remonstrated with him one evening when he had just removed the painting he had done in a hard day's work, saying he might have left it until the next morning. "No," he replied, "if I had left it till to-morrow I might have persuaded myself that it was good enough to leave permanently." The picture he had been working on was very interesting, and represented three girls in Japanese dress on a sort of terrace, one of them squatting on her heels while tending a plant in a pot. Another girl was standing and holding a parasol, which against the sky made an important mark in the composition. This dwells in my memory as one of the very best of Whistler's paintings. There was a version of it in the Whistler Exhibition at the New Gallery, but it lacked the quality of the former one. It may have been the old one repainted. This quality was to be seen in an oil sketch of it exhibited in Suffolk Street when Whistler was President of the Society of British Artists. I have always thought that at this time Whistler touched the highest point in his artistic career. I admit that he did many new things afterwards, such as his mother's portrait and the best of the Nocturnes and the Firework pictures, but he never again made the same sustained efforts. It was with reference to the Japanese subject that there was much talk of his making careful drawings of his figures, and cartoons which could be referred to as he was painting, so that he might not be worried about his drawing while he was intent on getting the best quality and colour in the surface of his paint. When living with Jameson in Great Russell Street, I think he did try this method while working on this very picture, but without success. It will be remembered by some that Albert Moore's influence with Whistler was very marked at this period.

Being so much absorbed in his methods, I worked in Whistler's manner on three or four occasions, and caught some of his quality. Two small heads I remember, and a dress of silk brocade, but I could never satisfy myself in this way in a whole picture. I had to retouch other parts, and so lost freshness of quality. The brocade dress I was very proud of, but when I came to the head of a very fair girl on the top of it, with honey-coloured hair in great quantity, I realized, if I had not known it before, how much more difficult it is to paint a human face than a piece of still-life.

Soon after our return to London Whistler and some of our friends used to paint still-life together at Poynter's studio in Grafton Street, and the results were interesting. This disciplinary practice is most valuable when carried out thoroughly, and with the exact relation of the foreground objects to their background well rendered. I have now one of these still-life studies done by Ridley at that time. He had been in Paris somewhat after the *Trilby* time, and had become intimate with Fantin and Legros. He was one of the most successful of Whistler's followers, and did some very good Thames pictures. The still-life piece referred to was done from some books, one of them opened lying on a table, with a drawing-board for a background. In fact just such a group of objects as was for many years prescribed by the Science and Art Department for disciplinary exercise in the Schools of Art. It has been the custom, however, for many years among writers on art to deride this method of study.

Fantin-Latour, it will be remembered by many, learnt a great deal as a painter by this practice, which can be carried on with the simplest materials and in the smallest room. He did not paint "d'emblée," that is, directly on to the bare canvas, after the Whistler fashion, but he drew and faintly modelled the composition with liquid oil-paint made of umber and white.

When Whistler showed the way, which he had learnt I suppose from Courbet, it seemed easy to carry the paint to a certain point of quality. I remember that one clever young fellow, Tom Morton, one of the ablest sketchers at the Langham Club, who had never been under such influence before, did some of these studies, which were accounted by the others as good as some done by their leader himself. It is not so very difficult to do a second- or third-rate Whistler, which would deceive the unwary.

Many years ago at the old Dudley Gallery there was an empty frame hanging on the wall, which was of a delicate grey tint, and somebody had, with charcoal, drawn an horizon on it, within the limit of the frame. With one or two spots judiciously placed, and perhaps the butterfly—though that may have been a later invention—it looked very like a Whistler from the other end of the gallery.

Some of the numerous writers about Whistler must have described his later methods of work. I do not know, for instance, how the best of the Firework pictures were done. The dark blue sea-piece which belonged to Mr. Rawlinson, and had to be repainted in consequence of the surface having decayed, was under-painted with a reddish-brown colour. John Chandler Bancroft, a great friend of mine and a devoted admirer of Whistler, said he saw it prepared with what he called a chocolate brown. The result, though not durable, was most successful in quality of colour. This method of under-painting with what would be called the complementary colour was written about by one Hundutpfund. I read his book as a boy, when I used to devour works on painting. That book and the account I had from Rome about the fancy methods of Page, the well-known American painter, led me into all kind of foolishness, to the neglect of the really serious work of drawing and direct painting, to which I ought to have been directing all my energies.

Fantin-Latour used to tell of a fad or pose of Whistler and some of his friends to use nothing but the simplest earth-colours, and to keep these in large pots covered with water, as is the custom of house-painters. They held at this time that the use of colours in tubes was in some way amateurish or effeminate; but, said Fantin, "if you looked carefully round the studio of one of these stalwarts, you would find hidden away in some corner a small paint-box containing the tubes of madder or the other tabooed paints, to be brought out for use when there was nobody about."

I remember Whistler telling me long afterwards, when he had been doing the studies of sunset skies on the coast of France, that he mixed and kept in pots a great number of tints more or less suitable for these evanescent effects. He could tell by experience a little time beforehand whether the evening sunset tints would be reddish or yellowish, and he prepared accordingly by selecting those mixed tints he was likely to want. From these, when the moment arrived for painting, he made other tints with but slight modifications, which took very little time. Some of these sky studies were very good indeed. I think the one bought by Frederick Jameson, the architect, was the most beautiful and desirable thing of the kind I remember. Whistler told du Maurier that he could copy any colour absolutely that he saw in Nature.

Doubtless an account has been written of Whistler's exhibition of etchings in Bond Street, a one-man show, as it would be called nowadays, which was got up by Sergeant Thomas in a shop by the Clarendon Hotel and nearly opposite Long's. I think it was a success, inasmuch as it made Jimmy's etched work known to the public for the first time.

Thomas was an eccentric old gentleman, a Serjeant-at-law (a rank at the English Bar which exists no longer), who used to frequent the studios of young artists and buy their pictures and sketches, sometimes paying for them in kind with a piece of furniture or bric-à-brac. I never heard anything against him except what Whistler said when the inevitable quarrel came. Jimmy had called to his aid a Greek lawyer, a very good fellow and clever, and the Greek and the Yankee brought all their forces to bear on the old lawyer.

There was a lively correspondence, and Whistler carried copies of his letters about in his pocket to read to any friends he came across. I am sure they were very clever and amusing, and I remember standing patiently at the corner of New Burlington Street while one or two of them were read to me. One day he read a letter he and his Greek partner had composed and despatched to the Serjeant, which they thought mighty clever and biting, and then he said: "There, that's what we sent him last, and what do you think? What does the old scoundrel do but die by return of post?" The epithet "scoundrel" was used only in the Pickwickian sense, I think.

I hardly ever knew any one who set such store by favourable newspaper criticisms as Whistler did. He had a friend who wrote for the Court Journal, and at the time of this exhibition Whistler treasured and carried about with him the favourable notices which had appeared in this paper, and had them out for perusal whenever he met a friend.

I have not looked up the file of The Times to see the terms in which Tom Taylor wrote about the first *At the Piano* exhibited at the Academy. But, as far as I can remember, it was a very generous recognition; indeed I have always thought that the virulent abuse Whistler and his later friends delighted in pouring on the Royal Academy must appear very misplaced and absurd to those who knew that his first picture, painted in an unaccustomed manner by an utterly unknown artist, who was besides a foreigner, was hung in a very good place on the line, and was bought before the exhibition opened by a Royal Academician, John Phillip.

We, his friends of that time, were amazed at his sudden and unexpected success, and gloried in it.

I remember preaching the gospel according to Saint Whistler to Tom Taylor one night as we returned together from a Greenwich dinner. It was an excellent and jovial dinner, and the famous art critic of those days was in a very good humour and listened patiently to my account of Jimmy's aims and his possible future. Shortly afterwards there was a laudatory notice of some of his work in The Times, but not nearly enough of it to satisfy me. Tom Taylor told du Maurier that he had written a great deal more which had been suppressed by the editor. This seemed to me very strange, for one would have thought that his position with regard to the paper was strong enough for him to insist on his article being printed as he wrote it. But Tom Taylor was a truthful person, and at that time very well-disposed.

I wonder if any of the numerous writers about the treatment of Whistler in this country have mentioned the fact that Mr. (afterwards Sir) Henry Cole let him have the use of a studio in the iron buildings put up temporarily to house the collections acquired for the Museum at South Kensington, and that he worked there for some time? The complaints so often made by his latest friends are to me incomprehensible. They knew well enough how free he was with his sharp tongue, and although in the early days he did not avowedly go out of the way to make enemies, his gibes at some of the most popular and commercially successful members of the Academy were enough to embitter them; besides, they did not understand or in any way sympathise with his work. We were amused, and applauded at the time—in the sixties—but it was quite natural and fair that those he attacked should retort as best they could. What a pity it was that the energy wasted in later years in "making enemies" was not spent on his painting.

I have often wished I could hear all Whistler had to say about his intercourse with Carlyle when the portrait was painted in 1872. He had a great many sittings for it, and there must have been much talk between them one would like to have heard repeated. I never learnt anything from Whistler's side, for at that time I had ceased to see him much, although there was no quarrel between us.

Allingham told us that Carlyle used always in speaking of Whistler to call him "The Creature." It seems very strange that two men so utterly different could have gone on so long in the close intercourse of the numerous sittings without friction enough to cause a break. For a long time Carlyle was not allowed to see the front of the canvas. He gave this account of his first sight of it: "At last, when he let me look at it,

I said, 'Oh, yes! I see, that is the mouth and that's the nose': but I was just told that all that was the beard, and that the face was somewhere up there," with a gesture.

I have been reading lately in a book about Whistler an account of his painting the room in Mr. Leyland's house in Prince's Gate, which became famous or notorious as the Peacock Room. There are few people if any now living who have accurate knowledge of what happened about this "teterrima belli causa." I will write down what little I remember about it. It was in 1876.

Tom Jeckyll, a very clever architect, and an early friend of du Maurier's before the Paris Trilby days, and afterwards well known to and much liked by the "Paris gang" when in London, was commissioned by Mr. Leyland to make a room suitable for housing his fine collection of blue and white oriental china. So he designed shelves or etagères with turned spindles or balusters to go round the room. The walls were to be covered with old Spanish or Dutch leather, of which a sufficient number of skins had been found and bought.

Jeckyll, who was quite abject in his admiration for Whistler, showed him the leather and asked his opinion as to its suitability. There were pink flowers in the pattern, and Jimmy suggested that these should be repainted with yellow; I think it was described as primrose colour. This alteration was obviously a happy one, having in view the purpose to which the leather was to be put, namely, to be a becoming background to the valuable blue china. When Whistler began to try the effect of repainting the flowers on the leather he found the surface agreeable to work on, and, disregarding the original pattern, he worked all over it and evolved the blue scheme which pleased him so much.

I was at that time predisposed to admire almost anything Whistler did, especially if he did not tell me it was very fine, as was often the case. The impression I received on seeing the room was not very favourable, for the colour did not serve as a happy background for people or furniture, and it was fatal to the precious blue china for the reception of which the alteration had been undertaken by Tom Jeckyll; the cobalt blue of the pots suffered terribly from juxtaposition with Whistler's paint, made of Prussian or Antwerp blue. It seemed to me a great pity to spoil the old leather, when it could easily have been removed and replaced by fresh and even canvas for Whistler to paint on. In my opinion the effect of the embossed pattern which showed through the paint was disturbing and unpleasant. I heard a great deal about the quarrel that ensued, but did not know anything at first-hand, and from Whistler's own account I sympathised with Mr. Leyland. I am afraid that Whistler in completely upsetting Jeckyll's scheme as he did brought about a crisis in his mental state, for he was lost sight of shortly afterwards. He was very clever in his profession and had many amiable qualities, but there had been perceptible for a long while a warp of eccentricity which at times suggested mental derangement.

I think I cannot have been in London when the trial Whistler *v.* Ruskin took place; at any rate I was not present in court. A little while before it came on I met Jimmy at the Arts Club, and he told me of his hopes with regard to the result, my sympathies being entirely on his side. I feared, however, that a jury could not be brought to see any beauties in Whistler's pictures, even the best of them, and therefore they might condone the brutality of Ruskin's attack. Whistler assured me, however, that he had evidence which must be effective in the shape of letters from Sir Frederick Leighton and Sir F. Burton, speaking highly of the "moonlight" pictures. These letters seemed to me most important, for they were written by people in official positions, a fact which would always weigh with the jurymen or ordinary bourgeois. Nothing was said about such letters in the newspaper reports of the trial, and when I asked Whistler the reason of this omission of the strongest evidence on his side, he told me that the writers of the letters had objected to their being put in, and therefore he had refrained from using them. The accounts he gave of the trial were very funny. He described the bewilderment of the jurymen as the paintings, the Nocturnes, were passed round for their inspection, and how, when Ruskin's Titian was brought in last of all, one of them exclaimed, "Now come, we've had enough of them Whistlers." He said it was handed to them upside down. When I saw Sir John Holker, who led for Ruskin, a fortnight afterwards and asked him if he had been helping to ruin any more poor artists, he said, "I was bound to do the best I could for my client." I objected to the production of the pictures in court, and he said he had insisted on it, so I told him I was sure he would not have allowed it if he had been Whistler's counsel. "Why didn't Jimmy have me?" he asked, and when I explained that I had recommended his being retained, but it was objected that his fee would be too high, he said: "I would have done it for nothing for Whistler." I was very sorry, for I do believe he would have won a very different verdict.

I know mention has been made of the legend Whistler put in chalk on the panel over the door of the White House in Tite Street on the morning of the day when the sale took place. He wrote, "Except the Lord build the house their labour is but vain that build it. E. W. Godwin built this one." But I do not think it has been told that an artist I knew in Chelsea, a devout and simple-minded man, came to the Arts Club that night and said he and his wife had been touched that morning at seeing from the writing in chalk over the door how ready Whistler was to acknowledge the hand of God in his recent misfortunes!

Whistler made many jokes at the expense

of his creditors which were current among his friends at the time of the débâcle at The White House, and these smart sayings have often been brought up against him as evidence of a want of moral sense. I don't think I liked them at the time, or afterwards, but then I knew that this kind of attitude towards creditors was part of the "programme." Did not Schaunard and Marcel aud Rodolphe in the *Vie de Bohême* always talk of creditors in that way? It was just as necessary for Whistler to take that line as it was for Huck Finn to carry out Tom Sawyer's programme.

I wonder if he ever told his friends in these late years the story of the creditor who saved him from drowning?

There was a tailor whom he had for a long time taken pains to avoid on account of unreasonable persistence in asking for payment of his bill. Jimmy had successfully kept out of his way and was thinking nothing about him, until once being in the water at one of the baths in the Seine he got out of his depth, and was struggling and spluttering in so desperate a way that the other bathers thought he would be drowned. One of them made a dash for him, caught him by his curls (which, as I have told you, were much longer in those days than he wore them during the last thirty years of his life) and dragged him to a place of safety. I can fancy how he looked with those long ringlets, their curliness straightened out, hanging over his face, and how when he had parted them and got the water out of his eyes he saw the face of his rescuer. It was that of his dunning tailor, into whose toils he had fallen through leaving dry land. Whistler told the story very well, as usual, and sheepishly admitted that he could not do less than pay the man after this rescue.

He was always known to us in Paris as James Abbott Whistler, and I think he signed " J. A. Whistler " until after his brother William came to England, when the American civil war was over. William had served as a doctor on the Confederate side, but Jimmy was always looked upon as a Yankee in his bringing-up and in his political views, if he had any.

Whistler once enquired from some relations of mine of the same name of the cradle of his race, and he was told that the Whistler family came from some place on a lake in Ireland; so he wrote to the incumbent of the parish for more information. In reply he was asked for a subscription towards the restoration of the church. The correspondence then came to an end.

Whistler's personal appearance was well known in London, though I do not remember having seen photographs of him in the shop windows.

I have one taken in Paris thirty years ago, or more, which gives a delightful and unaffected aspect of him. Both the powerful hands are well shown in it, those strong but delicate fingers which could lay on paint with such remarkable daintiness of touch, which at its best seemed unequalled.

One of the etched portraits of him by Mr. Mortimer Menpes is in my eyes a masterpiece, but there is something about it which is not altogether agreeable. I should have liked to do such a portrait of Jimmy after he had made a cruel joke at my expense, and was laughing loudly at it. What a pity it was that in later years he laughed so much and so loudly at his own good sayings, for thereby he spoiled much of the effect of them.

There was in the Whistler Exhibition at the New Gallery a painting he did of his own head and bust, which I saw in Lindsay Row soon after it was done. I admired it immensely, and have always considered it the best head I ever saw by him, but there was a little more to be done to it, and in attempting to do that little there was great risk of spoiling altogether the beautiful quality of the paint. He said he thought he might be able to retouch it, but was not sure. This was at the time when, as I have said before, he would take out all he had done in a day's work down to the clean canvas, if he did not think it good enough.

The portrait I saw in the New Gallery seemed to be the same, but if so, it had been spoiled by repainting. Not only was the paint of inferior quality, but there was a certain prettiness in the face which was neither characteristic nor agreeable. In its earlier state, if I am right in thinking it was the same canvas, the likeness was an excellent one, and agreeable—the good and pleasant side of Whistler. I am very sorry that the unfinished picture which I remember with so much pleasure was not preserved.

I wonder what has become of a caricature portrait of him which Pellegrini painted, to be used in a play at the Gaiety Theatre, in which there was a scene representing the studio of a very eccentric artist. It was an excellent performance, and if it is still in existence it ought to be taken care of. It was an oil-painting with the figure posed according to the manner of the "Whistlasquez" portraits, and was framed in the "Jimmy" style, the gold being tinted. For a long time it was on loan at the Arts Club, of which Pellegrini was a member and was to be seen there very often. The picture was not, to the best of my recollection, a spiteful caricature, and "Ape" was a great friend of Whistler's at that time. Is it necessary—perhaps it is—to tell you that Pellegrini was the clever Neapolitan who did the admirable caricatures signed "Ape" in Vanity Fair? He was a master in this kind of art, the best practising in this country I have known. I never saw much of him, but I liked him greatly, and I have carefully preserved some pencil sketches my friend Randolph Caldecott did of him on an envelope.

It pleased me not a little to hear from one who saw Whistler frequently till the end that he always spoke kindly of me, but I cannot take much credit to myself for never having had any quarrel or disagreement with him, for I had not seen him for some years before his death. We ceased to meet through living far apart and through my unwillingness to meet a man who was almost always with him at that time.

THE END.

PRINTED BY FRANCIS & CO
THE ATHENÆUM PRESS, 13, BREAM'S BUILDINGS,
LONDON, E C.

Printed in the USA
CPSIA information can be obtained
at www.ICGtesting.com
LVHW011521280823
756504LV00003B/52